S0-EYC-904
WITHDRAWN

Adequacy of the Comprehensive Clinical Evaluation Program

A Focused Assessment

Committee on the Evaluation of the Department of Defense Comprehensive Clinical Evaluation Program

Division of Health Promotion and Disease Prevention

INSTITUTE OF MEDICINE

NATIONAL ACADEMY PRESS
Washington, D.C. 1997

NATIONAL ACADEMY PRESS • 2101 Constitution Avenue, N.W. • Washington, DC 20418

NOTICE: The project that is the subject of this report was approved by the Governing Board of the National Research Council, whose members are drawn from the councils of the National Academy of Sciences, the National Academy of Engineering, and the Institute of Medicine. The members of the committee responsible for the report were chosen for their special competences and with regard for appropriate balance.

This report has been reviewed by a group other than the authors according to procedures approved by the Report Review Committee consisting of members of the National Academy of Sciences, the National Academy of Engineering, and the Institute of Medicine.

The Institute of Medicine was chartered in 1970 by the National Academy of Sciences to enlist distinguished members of appropriate professions in the examination of policy matters pertaining to the health of the public. In this, the Institute acts under both the Academy's 1863 congressional charter responsibility to be an adviser to the federal government and its own initiative in identifying issues of medical care, research, and education. Dr. Kenneth I. Shine is the president of the Institute of Medicine.

This study was supported by the US Department of Defense under Contract Number DASW01-96-K-007. The views presented are those of the Institute of Medicine Committee on the Evalution of the Department of Defense Comprehensive Clinical Evaluation Program and are not necessarily those of the funding organization.

International Standard Book No. 0-309-05949-6

Additional copies of this report are available for sale from:

National Academy Press
2101 Constitution Avenue, N.W.
Box 285
Washington, DC 20055

Call (800) 624-6242 or (202) 334-3313 (in the Washington metropolitan area), or visit the NAP's on-line bookstore at **http://www.nap.edu.**

For more information about the Institute of Medicine, visit the IOM home page at **http://www2.nas.edu/iom.**

Copyright 1997 by the National Academy of Sciences. All rights reserved.

Printed in the United States.

The serpent has been a symbol of long life, healing, and knowledge among almost all cultures and religions since the beginning of recorded history. The serpent adopted as a logotype by the Institute of Medicine is a relief carving from ancient Greece, now held by the Staatliche Museen in Berlin.

DS
79.744
.M44
A34
1997

WITHDRAWN

COMMITTEE ON THE EVALUATION OF THE DoD COMPREHENSIVE CLINICAL EVALUATION PROGRAM

Dan G. Blazer,* *Chair,* Dean of Medical Education and J.P. Gibbons Professor of Psychiatry, Duke University Medical Center, Durham, North Carolina

Rebecca Bascom, Director, Environmental Research Facility, University of Maryland, Baltimore

Margit L. Bleecker, Director of the Center for Occupational and Environmental Neurology, Baltimore, Maryland

Evelyn J. Bromet, Professor, Department of Psychiatry, State University of New York at Stony Brook, Stony Brook, New York

Gerard N. Burrow,* Special Advisor to the President for Health Affairs, Yale University School of Medicine, New Haven, Connecticut

Howard Kipen, Associate Professor and Chief, Occupational Health Division, UMDNJ, Robert Wood Johnson Medical School, Piscataway, New Jersey

Adel A. Mahmoud,* Chairman, Department of Medicine, Case Western Reserve University and University Hospitals of Cleveland, Cleveland, Ohio

Robert S. Pynoos, Professor of Psychiatry and Director of the Trauma Psychiatry Service, University of California, Los Angeles, California

Guthrie L. Turner, Jr., Chief Medical Consultant, Office of Disability Determination Services, State of Washington, Tummwater, Washington

Mark J. Utell, Professor of Medicine and Environmental Medicine and Director, Pulmonary/Critical Care and Occupational Medicine Divisions, University of Rochester Medical Center, Rochester, New York

Michael H. Weisman, Professor, Division of Rheumatology, Department of Medicine, University of California at San Diego

Board on Health Promotion and Disease Prevention Liaison

Elena O. Nightingale,* Scholar-in-Residence, Institute of Medicine and Board on Children, Youth and Families, Washington, DC

Board on Neuroscience and Behavioral Health Liaison

William E. Bunney, Jr.,* Distinguished Professor and Della Martin Chair of Psychiatry, University of California, Irvine, California

---

* Member, Institute of Medicine.

Staff

Lyla M. Hernandez, Study Director
Sanjay S. Baliga, Research Associate
Donna M. Livingston, Project Assistant
Kathleen R. Stratton, Director, Division of Health Promotion and Disease Prevention
Constance M. Pechura, Director, Division of Neuroscience and Behavioral Health
Donna D. Thompson, Division Assistant

Contents

Adequacy of the Comprehensive Clinical Evaluation Program

A Focused Assessment

Executive Summary

On August 2, 1990, Iraq invaded Kuwait. Within 5 days the United States had begun to deploy troops to the Persian Gulf in Operation Desert Shield. In January 1991, UN coalition forces began intense air attacks against the Iraqi forces (Operation Desert Storm), on February 24, a ground attack was launched and within 4 days, Iraqi resistance crumbled. Almost 700,000 US troops participated in the Persian Gulf War. Following the fighting, the number of US personnel began to decline rapidly.

Most troops returned home and resumed their normal activities. Within a relatively short time, a number of those who had been deployed to the Persian Gulf began to report health problems they believed to be connected to their deployment. These problems included the symptoms of fatigue, memory loss, severe headaches, muscle and joint pain, and rashes.

In 1992 the Department of Veterans Affairs (VA) developed a Persian Gulf Registry to assist in addressing questions about health concerns of Persian Gulf veterans. Exposures, particularly those associated with oil well fires, were included as part of the history taking. By 1994, with continuing concern about potential health consequences of service in the Persian Gulf, the Department of Defense (DoD) implemented a clinical evaluation program similar to the VA's and named it the Comprehensive Clinical Evaluation Program (CCEP).

Also in 1994, DoD asked the Institute of Medicine (IOM) to assemble a group of medical and public health experts to evaluate the adequacy of the CCEP. This committee concluded that although overall "the CCEP is a comprehensive effort to address the clinical needs of the thousands of active-duty personnel who served in the Gulf War," specific recommended changes in the protocol would help to increase its diagnostic yield. (See Appendix D for a complete set of recommendations.)

Late in 1995, DoD asked the IOM to continue its evaluation of the CCEP with special attention to the adequacy of the protocol as it related to (1) difficult-to-diagnose individuals and those with ill-defined conditions; (2) the diagnosis and treatment of patients with stress and psychiatric conditions; and (3) assessment of the health problems of those who may have been exposed to low levels of nerve agents. It is important to note what was not included in the committee charge. It was *not* the committee's charge to determine whether or not there is such an entity (or entities) as "Persian Gulf Illness" nor was it this committee's charge to determine whether or not there are long-term health effects from low-level exposure to nerve agents. These questions are more properly the subject for extensive scientific research.

Given the urgency surrounding the last question—the health problems of individuals with possible exposure to low levels of nerve agents—the committee addressed this issue first and separately, releasing its report, *Adequacy of the Comprehensive Clinical Evaluation Program: Nerve Agents,* in April 1997. The committee concluded that although the CCEP continues to provide an appropriate screening approach to the diagnosis of disease, certain refinements would enhance its value. A complete set of recommendations is found in Appendix F.

To complete the remaining portions of its charge, the committee convened two workshops on the relevant topics, heard presentations, reviewed written material, and received comments from leading scientific and clinical experts, representatives of DoD and the VA, the Presidential Advisory Committee, the General Accounting Office, and representatives of veterans groups.

A great deal of time and effort has been expended evaluating DoD's Comprehensive Clinical Evaluation Program. It has been reviewed by the President's Advisory Committee, the General Accounting Office, the Office of Technology Assessment, the Institute of Medicine, and many other organizations. As more is learned, it becomes easier to focus on the kinds of questions the CCEP should be asking. As Dr. Penelope Keyl said in her workshop presentation on the development of good screening instruments, progress made over time will necessitate new generations of screening instruments. This does not imply that the first instrument developed is bad, but rather that time leads to new knowledge, which leads to the ability to improve the instrument.

Such is the case with the CCEP. Over time, the CCEP and other programs have generated information that has increased our understanding and led us to focus on areas of importance for those concerned about the health consequences of Persian Gulf deployment. This information has enabled us to take a closer look, to make a more thorough examination of the system, and to identify areas in which change will be of benefit. The committee believes that such change is healthy, that it reflects growth, and that it should be a natural part of any system having as one of its goals the delivery of high-quality health care services.

Change also occurs with individuals. It may be that as time passes or new information is released, some of those who have already participated in the CCEP will develop new concerns or problems. The committee hopes that DoD will encourage these individuals to return to the CCEP for further evaluation and diagnosis if they so desire.

CONCLUSIONS AND RECOMMENDATIONS

Medically Unexplained Symptom Syndromes

The committee spent time deliberating on the precise meaning of "difficult to diagnose" or "ill defined" as a description of a category of conditions. Difficult to diagnose is generally used to describe a condition for which special expertise is required to arrive at a diagnosis, but some of the conditions under consideration do not require such expertise. Chronic fatigue syndrome (CFS), fibromyalgia, and multiple chemical sensitivity are symptom complexes that have a great deal of overlap in the symptoms present in each condition. They are symptom-based, without objective findings. However, they are actually fairly well defined by operational criteria, even if they are medically unexplained. Despite the fact that they are medically unexplained, they may cause significant impairment, and they are conditions that are better understood through time (i.e., adequate evaluation of these disorders requires a longitudinal perspective that includes knowledge of previous services and responses to treatment). The committee decided, therefore, to refer to this spectrum of illnesses as *medically unexplained symptom syndromes.* This spectrum of illnesses may include those which are etiologically unexplained, lack currently detectable pathophysiological changes, and/or cannot currently be diagnostically labeled.

Medically unexplained symptom syndromes are often associated with depression and anxiety, yet this does not imply that the syndromes are psychiatric disorders. There remains a debate about how to distinguish these syndromes from psychiatric diagnoses. However, since most of the recommended treatments for medically unexplained symptom syndromes overlap with the pharmacological and behavioral treatments for psychiatric diagnoses, the committee believes that it is important to identify and evaluate the symptoms associated with these conditions and then treat those symptoms.

- **The committee recommends that when patients presenting with medically unexplained symptom syndromes are evaluated, the provider**

must have access to the full and complete medical record, including previous use of services.

In the area of medically unexplained symptom syndromes, it is sometimes not possible to arrive at a definitive diagnosis. It may be possible, however, to treat the presenting complaints or symptoms.

- **The committee recommends that in cases where a diagnosis cannot be identified, treatment should be targeted to specific symptoms or syndromes (e.g., fatigue, pain, depression).**
- **The committee recommends that the CCEP be encouraged to identify patients in this spectrum of illnesses early in the process of their disease. In addition, primary care providers should identify the patients' functional impairments so as to be able to suggest treatments that will assist in improving these disabilities.**

Stress

Stress is a major issue in the lives of patients within this spectrum of illness. Stress need not be looked at so much as a causative agent, but rather as a part of the condition of the patient that cannot be ignored. With medically unexplained symptom syndromes, the potential for stress proliferation is great among both the person deployed to the Persian Gulf and the family members.

Research has shown that stressors have been associated with major depression, substance abuse, and various physical health problems. Those deployed to the Gulf were exposed to a vast array of different stressors that carry with them their own potential health consequences. The current collection of exposure information does not adequately address an investigation of traumatic events to which the deployed soldier may have been exposed. In addition, media attention and reports by the military to Gulf War veterans that toxic exposure could have occurred are very stressful events. The stress associated with these reports needs to be recognized and addressed.

- **The committee recommends that the CCEP contain questions on traumatic event exposures in addition to the exposure information currently being collected. This would include the addition of open-ended questions that ask the patient to list the events that were most upsetting to him or her while deployed. Positive responses to questions regarding such events, as well as to other exposure questions, should be pursued with a *narrative inquiry*, which would address such items as the specific nature of the exposure; the duration; the frequency of repetition; the dose or**

intensity (if appropriate); whether the patient was taking protective measures and, if so, what these measures were; and the symptoms manifested.

- **The committee recommends that DoD providers acknowledge stressors as a legitimate but not necessarily sole cause of physical symptoms and conditions.**

Every soldier who goes to war will be subjected to major disturbing events since war involves death and destruction. There are certain jobs undertaken in the midst of war that, by their very nature, result in high stress (e.g., grave registration duty). The effect of stress associated with these jobs can be mitigated if approached properly. Such efforts, however, require time for the provider and the patient to interact. It is not possible to hand the patient a pamphlet or a questionnaire and expect that all necessary information will be revealed or understood.

- **The committee recommends that DoD provide special training and debriefing for those who are engaged in high-risk jobs such as jobs associated with the Persian Gulf experience.**
- **The committee recommends that DoD provide to each about-to-be deployed soldier, risk or hazard communication that is well developed and designed to provide information regarding what the individual can expect and the potentially traumatic events to which he or she might be exposed.**
- **The committee recommends that adequate time must be provided during initial interactions with patients in the CCEP in order to insure that all pertinent information is forthcoming.**

Screening

Depression is a condition that is common in primary care. Most individuals who experience depression continue to function, but if they are left untreated, their condition may deteriorate. Unlike many of the medically unexplained symptom syndromes, there are accepted and effective treatments for depression.

- **The committee recommends that there be increased screening at the primary care level for depression.**
- **Every primary care physician should have a simple standardized screen for depression. If a patient scores in the significant range, this person should be referred to a qualified mental health professional for further evaluation and treatment.**
- **If depression is identified, there has to be more questioning on exposure to traumatic situations.**

- **The committee recommends that any individual who reports any significant symptoms of posttraumatic stress disorder (PTSD) and/or a significant traumatic stressor should be referred to a qualified mental health professional for further evaluation and treatment.**

Substance abuse or misuse problems are prevalent in primary care. In addition, individuals under stress and/or with untreated depression or medically unexplained symptom syndromes may be at increased risk for substance abuse.

- **The committee recommends that every primary care physician have a simple, standardized screen for substance abuse. Every individual who screens positive should be referred for further evaluation and treatment.**

There are certain areas in which baseline assessments are of immense value in the clinical evaluation of an individual patient's status (e.g., pulmonary function and neurobehavioral testing). Changes in neurocognitive and peripheral nerve function are measured by comparing the individual's current status to a baseline measure. Individual baseline information is necessary because the variability across individuals is too great to identify a generalized "normal" screening level.

- **The committee recommends that DoD explore the possibility of using neurobehavioral testing at entry into the military to determine whether it is feasible to use such tests to predict change in functioning or track change in function during a soldier's military career.**

Program Evaluation

Most patients in the CCEP receive a diagnosis after completing a Phase I examination; some are referred to Phase II for evaluation; and a few have gone on to participate in the program at the Specialized Care Center (SCC). Information presented to the committee indicates that there is great variation across regions in the percentage of patients who are diagnosed with primary psychiatric diagnoses and medically unexplained symptom syndromes. A determination should be made as to why this variation exists. Although there may be many reasons, one explanation could relate to the consistency with which procedures for diagnosis and referral are implemented from facility to facility.

- **The committee recommends that an evaluation be conducted to examine (1) the consistency with which Phase I examinations are conducted across facilities; (2) the patterns of referral from Phase I to Phase II; and**

(3) the adequacy of treatment provided to certain categories of patients where there is the potential for great impact on patient outcomes when effective treatment is rendered (e.g., depression).

The SCC has provided evaluation and treatment to 78 patients since it was begun. A great deal of effort and thought has gone into the development of a program designed to help the patient understand his or her conditions and engage in behaviors most likely to result in improvement. The committee was asked to assess the effectiveness of this center, but realized that such an assessment depended on a number of factors that have not been well defined. What is the goal of the center—is it treatment, research, or education? Should a major consideration in the center's evaluation be cost-effectiveness? Should the numbers of those receiving care be taken into consideration and, if so, what are the barriers to patients accessing this level of care? What is the triage process by which individuals get referred to the SCC?

- **The committee recommends that a short-term (perhaps 5-year) plan be developed for the Specialized Care Center that would specify goals and expected outcomes.**

Coordination with the VA

Given that many now receiving services in the DoD health care system will eventually move to the VA health care system, it is important for there to be good communication between DoD and the VA. This may be particularly true in the areas of medically unexplained symptom syndromes and psychiatric disorders, where accurate diagnosis and/or assessment of response to treatment is important for positive patient outcomes.

- **The committee recommends that DoD explore ways to increase communication with the VA, particularly as it relates to the ongoing treatment of patients.**

Both providers and patients would benefit from increased educational activity regarding Persian Gulf health issues. Provider turnover within DoD is a factor that must be taken into consideration when examining the special health needs and concerns of active-duty personnel who were deployed to the Persian Gulf. Although efforts to educate providers were extensive at the time the CCEP was implemented, 3 years have passed and many new providers have entered the system. These individuals should be oriented to the special needs, concerns, and procedures involved, and all providers should be updated regularly.

The VA has developed a number of approaches to provider education which could serve as useful models. Interactive satellite teleconferences are available for medical center staff to discuss particular issues of concern. The VA conducts quarterly national telephone conference calls, directs periodic educational mailings to Persian Gulf Registry providers in each health facility, and conducts an annual conference on the health consequences of Persian Gulf service.

In addition to providers, there is a great need for education of and communication with individuals (and their families) who were deployed to the Gulf. These individuals are concerned about the potential impact of Persian Gulf deployment on their health, whether or not their health concerns will affect their military careers, their ability to obtain health insurance once they leave the service, and a number of other issues that need to be addressed.

- **The committee recommends that DoD examine the activities and materials for provider education developed by the VA to determine if some of the items might be used as educational approaches for DoD providers.**
- **The committee recommends that DoD mount an effort designed to educate providers to the fact that conditions related to stress are not necessarily psychiatric conditions. The committee recommends that depression be a topic of education for all primary care providers, with emphasis on the facts that depression is common, it is treatable, and individuals who experience depression can continue to function.**
- **The committee recommends that CCEP information be used to develop case studies that will help educate providers about Persian Gulf health problems.**
- **The committee recommends that DoD develop approaches to communication and education that address the concerns of individuals deployed to the Persian Gulf and their families.**

Determining the etiology(ies) of health problems experienced by those deployed to the Persian Gulf War may not always be possible. However, it is possible that treatment can be provided for many of the symptoms or conditions associated with some of these problems. The committee wishes, therefore, to emphasize the importance of adequate assessment of medically unexplained symptom syndromes and of traumatic event exposure, as well as screening for depression and for substance abuse. Such additions to the CCEP will enhance its ability to identify and, ultimately, treat the health problems being experienced by those who served in the Persian Gulf War.

Table 1 provides a summary of the committee's recommendations.

TABLE 1 Summary of Committee Recommendations

Topic	Recommendation
Medically unexplained symptom syndromes	• The provider evaluating these patients must have access to the complete medical record including prior treatment. • Rather than attempting to fit a treatment to a diagnosis, treatment should target specific symptoms or syndromes (e.g., pain, fatigue, depression). • A patient's functional impairments should be identified early to facilitate treatment.
Stress	• The initial CCEP examination should include questions regarding traumatic event exposure. Any positive response should be followed up with a narrative inquiry. • Stressors must be acknowledged as a legitimate but not necessarily sole cause of physical symptoms and conditions. • DoD should provide special training and debriefing for those engaged in high-risk jobs during deployment, e.g., graves registration. • DoD should provide risk or hazard communication to each about-to-be deployed soldier. • Adequate time must be provided for provider/patient interaction during CCEP examinations.
Screening	• There should be increased screening for depression at the primary care level. • Every physician should employ a simple, standardized screen for depression (e.g., BDI, Zung Scale, CES-D, IDD). • Patients who screen positive for depression should be referred for screening, further evaluation, and treatment. • Patients diagnosed with depression should be interviewed regarding traumatic exposure. • Patients identified with any significant PTSD symptoms and/or a significant traumatic stressor should be referred to a qualified mental health professional for further evaluation and treatment. • Every physician should employ a simple standardized screen for substance abuse (e.g., CAGE, brief MAST, T-ACE, TWEAK, AUDIT). • Every patient who screens positive for substance abuse should be referred for further evaluation and treatment. • DoD should explore feasibility of neurobehavioral testing at entry into military for usefulness in measuring change in function.

Continued

TABLE 1 *Continued*

Topic	Recommendation
Program evaluation	• An evaluation should be conducted to examine: (1) the consistency of Phase I examinations across facilities; (2) the patterns of referral program from Phase I to Phase II; and (3) the adequacy of treatment provided to certain categories of patients where the potential for positive impact is great (e.g., depression). • DoD should develop a short-term plan for the Specialized Care Center that specifies goals and expected outcomes.
Education	• DoD should explore ways to increase communication with the VA, particularly as it relates to the ongoing treatment of patients. • DoD should examine the provider education materials and programs developed by the VA to determine if they might serve as models for DoD approaches. • Education is needed to emphasize that conditions related to stress are not necessarily psychiatric conditions. • Education should emphasize that depression is common and treatable, and that patients with depression can continue to function. • CCEP information should be used to develop case studies which will help educate providers about Persian Gulf health problems. • DoD educational efforts should also address the concerns of Persian Gulf-deployed individuals and their families.

1

Introduction

A large Iraqi force invaded the independent nation of Kuwait on August 2, 1990. Within 5 days, in response to United Nations Resolution 678, the United States began deploying troops to the Persian Gulf in Operation Desert Shield. On January 16, 1991, UN coalition forces began intense air attacks against the Iraqi forces (Operation Desert Storm). By February 1991, more than 500,000 US troops were present and ready to engage the Iraqi army. A ground attack was launched on February 24, and within 4 days Iraqi resistance crumbled. After the fighting, the number of US troops in the area began to decline rapidly. By June 1991, fewer than 50,000 US troops remained.

Almost 700,000 US troops participated in Operations Desert Shield and Desert Storm. The composition of these troops differed from any previous US armed force. Overall, they were older; a large proportion (about 17%) were from National Guard and Reserve units; and almost 7% of the total forces were women.

The US casualties were low during the Persian Gulf War. There were 148 combat deaths, with an additional 145 deaths due to disease or accident. Despite the low number of fatalities and injuries, service personnel in the Persian Gulf were exposed to a number of stressors. These included environmental factors such as oil smoke, diesel and jet fuel, solvents and other petrochemicals, CARC (chemical agent resistant coating) paint, depleted uranium, chemical warfare agents, sand, and endemic infections such as leishmaniasis. In addition, some soldiers were given anthrax and botulinum vaccines and ingested pyridostigmine bromide pills to protect against chemical warfare agents.

Other stressors included the rapid mobilization for military service, with an accompanying disruption of normal patterns; the unfamiliar character of the region and the requirement that US military personnel have virtually no interaction with the indigenous populations; the primitive living conditions of US troops; and the immense destruction visited on the whole nation of Iraq.

After the war, most troops returned home and resumed their normal activities. Within a relatively short time, a number of active-duty military personnel and veterans reported various health problems that they believed were connected to their Persian Gulf deployment. Symptoms commonly described include fatigue, memory loss, severe headaches, muscle and joint pain, and rashes (Schwarts et al., 1997). As reports of a purported "Persian Gulf illness" circulated, public concern grew.

In 1992, the Department of Veterans Affairs (VA) developed and implemented the Persian Gulf Registry to create a mechanism for tracking medical and other data on Persian Gulf veterans. It was thought that information in the Registry would assist in addressing questions about possible future effects of exposure to air pollutants and other environmental agents. In addition, this Registry was to serve as the basis for future medical surveillance of Persian Gulf veterans. Exposures, particularly those associated with the oil well fires, were included as part of the history taking.

As concern continued to escalate, the Department of Defense (DoD) also decided to develop and implement a Persian Gulf clinical program. DoD and the VA met, used experts to develop clinical protocols, and by 1994, had implemented similar clinical evaluation programs. DoD named its program the Comprehensive Clinical Evaluation Program (CCEP). The stated purpose of the CCEP is to diagnose and treat active-duty military personnel who have medical complaints that they attribute to service in the Gulf.

In addition to the clinical programs, research investigations were launched to discover whether or not there is such an entity (or entities) as Persian Gulf illness. Other examinations of Persian Gulf issues and the government's response were undertaken by the General Accounting Office and the Office of Technology Assessment. In May 1995, President Clinton announced the establishment of a Presidential Advisory Committee on Gulf War Veterans' Illnesses. This Advisory Committee was charged with analyzing the government's coordination and activities regarding outreach, medical care, research, and chemical and biological weapons, pertinent to Gulf War veterans' illnesses. It also investigated the short- and long-term health effects of Gulf War risk factors.

The Presidential Advisory Committee report, released on December 31, 1996, concluded that it is vital to continue to provide clinical care to evaluate and treat the illnesses that many veterans are clearly experiencing in connection with their service in the Gulf War. The Advisory Committee *did not*, however, discover any research or evidence documenting a causal link between any single factor and the symptoms reported by Gulf War veterans. Although several recommendations were made to "fine-tune" the government's programs on Gulf War health matters, the Advisory Committee concluded that only in the area of DoD's efforts related to chemical weapons were there serious questions. For a complete set of Presidential Advisory Committee recommendations, see Appendix A.

2

Overview of the Institute of Medicine's Persian Gulf Activities

The Institute of Medicine (IOM) has undertaken several activities focusing on the potential health implications of deployment in the Persian Gulf War and the efforts of DoD and the VA to respond to health concerns. The IOM Medical Follow-up Agency conducted a project focused on the health consequences of service in the Gulf and developed recommendations for research and information systems. The first report of this group (IOM, 1995b) concluded that there had been a fragmented attempt to solve the health problems of Persian Gulf veterans and that "sustained, coordinated, and serious efforts must be made in the near term to focus both the medical, social, and research response of the Government and of individuals and researchers." (See Appendix B for a complete set of recommendations.) The second report of the Medical Follow-up Agency (IOM, 1996b) detailed 16 recommendations with accompanying findings concerning research and information systems needed regarding the health consequences of service during the Persian Gulf War (Appendix C).

In 1994, DoD asked the IOM to assemble a group of medical and public health experts to evaluate the adequacy of the CCEP. The first committee met four times and prepared three reports between October 1994 and January 1996 (IOM, 1994, 1995a, 1996a). The committee concluded that although overall "the CCEP is a comprehensive effort to address the clinical needs of the thousands of active-duty personnel who served in the Gulf War," specific recommended changes in the protocol would help to increase its diagnostic yield. The committee also concluded that the CCEP is *not* appropriate as a research tool but that the results could and should be used to educate Persian Gulf veterans and the physicians caring for them, to improve the medical protocol itself, and to evaluate patient outcomes. A complete list of the first CCEP committee's recommendations appears in Appendix D.

Late in 1995, DoD asked the IOM to continue its evaluation of the CCEP with special attention to three issues: (1) difficult-to-diagnose individuals and those with ill-defined conditions; (2) the diagnosis and treatment of patients with stress and psychiatric conditions; and (3) assessment of the health problems of those who may have been exposed to low levels of nerve agents. The committee was also to consider whether there are medical tests or consultations that should be added systematically to the CCEP to increase its diagnostic yield. A new committee was convened to address these issues. Most members of the newly formed committee were also members of the first IOM CCEP committee.

In defining the tasks included in this review, the committee noted what was *not* included in its charge. It was *not* this committee's charge to determine whether there is such an entity (or entities) as Persian Gulf Illness, nor was it this committee's charge to determine whether there are long-term health effects from low-level exposure to nerve agents. These questions are more properly the subject of extensive scientific research.

A series of workshops was planned to obtain information on these topics. Given the urgency surrounding the question of health problems of those who may have been exposed to low levels of nerve agents, DoD asked the committee to address this topic first, separately and as rapidly as possible. A 1-day workshop was held on December 3, 1996, during which information was gathered from leading researchers and clinicians about the effects of exposure to nerve agents and chemically related compounds, as well as about tests available to measure the potential health effects of such exposures. (See Appendix E for the workshop agenda and list of participants.)

The committee reviewed extensive clinical and research results regarding the effects of nerve agents, including those presented at the workshop as well as in the literature. In its report *Adequacy of the Comprehensive Clinical Evaluation Program: Nerve Agents* (1997), the committee concluded that although the CCEP continues to provide an appropriate screening approach to the diagnosis of disease, certain refinements would enhance its value. For a complete set of recommendations, see Appendix F.

Over the course of the project, the committee heard presentations, reviewed written material, and received comments from leading scientific and clinical experts; representatives of the Department of Defense and the Department of Veterans Affairs; the Presidential Advisory Committee; the General Accounting Office; and representatives of veterans' groups. The committee also held two public workshops (see Appendix G for workshop agendas and participant lists).

3

The Comprehensive Clinical Evaluation Program*

OVERVIEW

In June 1994, DoD instituted the CCEP to provide a thorough, systematic clinical evaluation program for the diagnosis and treatment of Persian Gulf veterans at military facilities in the US and overseas.

The CCEP was designed to (1) strengthen the coordination between DoD and the VA; (2) streamline patient access to medical care; (3) make clinical diagnoses in order to treat patients; (4) provide a standardized, staged evaluation and treatment program; and (5) assess possible Gulf War-related conditions. (Veterans who have left military service entirely are eligible for evaluations from the VA; personnel still on active duty, in the Reserves, or in the National Guard may request medical evaluations from DoD.) Phase I of the CCEP consists of a medical history, physical examinations, and laboratory tests. These are comparable in scope and thoroughness to an evaluation conducted during an inpatient internal medicine hospital admission (see Appendix H). All CCEP participants are evaluated by a primary care physician at their local medical treatment facility and receive specialty consultations if these are deemed appropriate by their primary care physician. Evaluation at this phase includes a survey for nonspecific patient symptoms, including fatigue, joint pain, diarrhea, difficulty concentrating, memory and sleep disturbances, and rashes.

---

*The material in this section is based, in part, on presentations and discussion by Lt. Col. Tim Cooper, M.D., MAJ Charles Engel, M.D., COL Kurt Kroenke, M.D., MAJ Charles Magruder, M.D., and MAJ Michael Roy, M.D.

The primary care physician may refer patients to Phase II for further specialty consultations if he or she determines that it is clinically indicated. These Phase II evaluations are conducted at a regional medical center and consist of targeted, symptom-specific examinations, lab tests, and consultations. During this phase, the potential causes of unexplained illnesses are assessed, including infectious agents, environmental exposures, social and psychological factors, and vaccines or other protective agents. Both Phase I and Phase II are intended to be thorough for each individual patient and to be consistent among patients.

Every medical treatment facility has a designated CCEP physician coordinator who is a board-certified family practitioner or internal medicine specialist. The coordinator is responsible for overseeing both the comprehensiveness and the quality of Phase I exams. At regional medical centers, CCEP activities are coordinated by board-certified internal medicine specialists who also oversee program operations of the medical treatment facilities in their region.

In March 1995, DoD established the Specialized Care Center at Walter Reed Army Medical Center to provide additional evaluation, treatment, and rehabilitation for patients who are suffering from chronic debilitating symptoms. Seventy-eight patients have gone through the Specialized Care Program, which consists of an intensive 3-week evaluation and treatment protocol designed to improve their health status.

The Specialized Care Center has three teams that overlap: (1) the physical team (physiatrist, physical therapist, occupational therapist, fitness trainer); (2) the medical team (internist, physiatrist, specialists, nutritionist); and (3) the psychosocial team (psychologist, social worker, wellness coordinator). Physical training, individualized to the patient, is an important part of the program, as is education. The program works with the patient on issues that result in dysfunction or impairment. The focus is not on the cause of the problems, but rather on how the patient can get better.

SIGNS, SYMPTOMS, AND ILL-DEFINED CONDITIONS (SSID)

The Department of Defense reported to the committee that approximately 17% of the 21,579 patients in the CCEP had a primary diagnosis of SSID, while about 42% had "any diagnosis" of SSID. The subcategories of SSID are symptoms, nonspecific abnormal findings, and ill-defined and unknown causes of morbidity and mortality. Of the patients with SSID, 96.6% (3,591 patients) of the diagnoses were in the symptom subcategory, 3% (112) in the nonspecific abnormal finding subcategory, and 0.4% (16) in the remaining subcategory (Table 3.1).

TABLE 3.1 Diagnoses Within the Symptom Group (percentage)

Symptom	Primary Diagnosis	Any Diagnosis
Fatigue	27	30
Sleep disturbance	18	24
Headache	14	21
Memory loss	10	16
Chest pain	5	7
Rash	4	5

DoD reported that a comparison of patients in the diagnostic categories of primary SSID, any SSID, non-SSID, and healthy found essentially no differences in percentages of males and females, no significant age differences, and no significant ethnic differences. For branch of service, the Marines are slightly more represented in the non-SSID population. In a comparison of active-duty versus reserve status, the active duty are slightly more likely to be in the non-SSID diagnostic category, whereas the reserves are slightly more likely to be in an SSID category (Table 3.2).

TABLE 3.2 Most Common Primary SSID Diagnosis by Phase of CCEP (percentage)

Symptom	Phase I	Phase II
Fatigue	28	18.0
Sleep disturbance	17	37.5
Headache	14	17.0
Memory loss	10	6.5
Chest pain	5	2.5
Rash	4	1.5

Of the 21,579 patients seen in Phase I, 4,012 (18.6%) initially received an SSID diagnosis. Of these, 703 (17.5%) were referred to Phase II; only 239 (34%) of this group continued to be diagnosed with SSID, whereas 464 (66%) received an alternative diagnosis that did not include SSID. About 40% of these changed to a primary diagnosis within the psychological category. However, 3,309 patients who received an SSID diagnosis at Phase I were not referred to Phase II.

Of the 17,567 patients who did not receive a diagnosis of SSID, 1,603 were referred for a Phase II exam. Of these, 171 received an SSID diagnosis, whereas 1,432 had no SSID diagnosis assigned. In summary, DoD reported no demographic differences between SSID and non-SSID patients; fatigue is the most common chief complaint in SSID patients; joint pain is the most common chief complaint in non-SSID patients; the most common primary SSID diagnosis differs by phase; and a diagnosis of primary SSID made in Phase I is commonly changed in Phase II.

CHRONIC FATIGUE SYNDROME (CFS) AND FIBROMYALGIA IN THE CCEP POPULATION

The Centers for Disease Control and Prevention (CDC) consensus definition for CFS and the American College of Rheumatology (ACR) definition of fibromyalgia were communicated to all medical treatment facilities in March 1995. Those performing Phase I and Phase II examinations were encouraged to use these definitions.

Of the total population seen in the CCEP, 12.4%, or 3,078, individuals received any diagnosis of fatigue (ICD-9 780.7). A **primary** diagnosis of fatigue was given to 4.5%, or 1,120 individuals. Of the 1,120 individuals receiving a primary diagnosis of fatigue, 48 (4%) were diagnosed with CFS, 8 (1%) with idiopathic chronic fatigue, 242 (22%) with chronic fatigue, and 822 (73%) with fatigue. If **secondary** diagnoses are included, a total of 74 individuals received a diagnosis of CFS. Thus, CFS was diagnosied in 2.4% of the population who received any diagnosis of fatigue but only in 0.3% of the total 24, 823[1] CCEP participants.

The prevalence of CFS in the general population ranges from 0.007% to 0.037%; in medical clinics, from 0.13% to 0.3%, and in fatigue clinics it is 5.0%. For fibromyalgia, according to the ACR definition, of the 24,823 CCEP participants, 141 (0.57%) had a primary diagnosis of fibromyalgia and an additional 177 (0.71%) had any secondary diagnosis of fibromyalgia. For the total number (318) of patients with either a primary or a secondary diagnosis of fibromyalgia, the number of patients with the comorbid diagnoses are shown in Table 3.3.

---

[1]Individuals within DoD conducted analyses of CCEP data based on committee requests for information; therefore, these analyses were performed at different times. As a result, the total number of CCEP participants varied. Analysis of SSID was conducted on a total CCEP population of 21,579 patients, whereas analysis of CFS and fibromyalgia included 24,823 CCEP participants. Since the committee focused not on numbers of cases but rather on general patterns, members did not feel it was necessary to ask for updated figures.

TABLE 3.3 Number of Comorbid Diagnoses in Patients with Primary or Secondary Diagnosis of Fibromyalgia

Irritable bowel syndrome	57 (17.9%)
Tension headaches	44 (13.8%)
Sleep disturbances	65 (20.4%)
Depression	77 (24.2%)
Posttraumatic stress disorder	54 (17.0%)

Table 3.4 shows the symptoms associated with CFS and fibromyalgia. The first column lists the symptom; the CCEP column refers to the percentage of CCEP patients complaining of that symptom; the fibromyalgia and CFS columns represent percentages of patients diagnosed with these conditions who complain of that symptom.

TABLE 3.4 Percentage of Patients Diagnosed with the Condition They Complain About

Sympton	CCEP (%)	Fibro (%)	CFS (%)
Difficulty concentrating	26.8	53.8	59.5
Headache	39.6	60.4	55.4
Joint pain	51.2	76.4	68.9
Memory deficit	34.6	59.7	62.2
Muscle pain	21.8	62.3	44.6
Sleep disturbance	33.6	60.7	52.7
Abdominal pain	16.4	36.2	28.4
Bleeding gums	8.5	18.6	12.2
Depression	22.1	46.9	45.9
Diarrhea	22.1	46.9	45.9
Hair loss	12.5	17.9	14.9
Rash	29.9	40.6	50.0
Dyspnea	19.2	29.9	32.4

STRESS AND PSYCHIATRIC DISORDERS

Patients who are referred to Phase II are much more likely to receive a psychological diagnosis than those who are diagnosed in Phase I. It is also the case that psychological diagnoses seem to be more common in the enlisted population. In looking at the prevalence of psychological diagnoses, whether primary or secondary, somatoform disorders account for 14.3% and mood disorders for 12.8%. The prevalence of posttraumatic stress disorder (PTSD) is 5.5%; anxiety disorders, 3.2%; substance abuse, 4.2%; and other psychological diagnoses, 8.5%.

Mood disorders and PTSD are almost equally likely to be primary or secondary, whereas somatoform disorders, substance abuse, and other anxiety disorders are much more likely to be secondary diagnoses. In examining the distribution of primary psychological diagnoses over time, it has been found that depression increased from about one-third of the diagnoses in the last half of 1994 to almost 50% of the primary psychological diagnoses in the last half of 1996, with the greatest portion of this increase occurring in the last 6 months. Depression is also more common among older patients.

Women are more likely to be diagnosed with somatoform and mood disorders, whereas PTSD and substance abuse are more common among men. In terms of duty status, mood disorders and PTSD tend to be more common among guards or reservists and retired participants than among those on active duty, whereas somatoform disorders are more common among the active-duty population (Table 3.5).

If tension headache is included as a somatoform disorder, it is by far the most common at 19.4% of the 24.6% with a primary diagnosis of somatoform disorder. For those with a primary diagnosis of substance abuse, the most common disorder is generally alcohol misuse followed by misuse of tobacco. Any other substance abuse problems were distinctly rare, with only 4 individuals (0.1%) in this category.

For those in the category of primary other psychiatric diagnosis, 7.9% are adjustment disorders and 3.7% organic mental disorders (*Note*: some of these are reported as actually being psychosis due to alcohol or substance abuse); sleep disorders represent 3.2%; schizophrenia or unspecified psychosis amount to 0.2%, and other disorders constitute 2.5%.

For the 7,564 individuals who received a secondary psychiatric diagnosis, the most common diagnosis was somatoform disorders (39.2%) followed by mood disorders (26.9%), substance abuse (14.1%), PTSD (11%), anxiety disorders (8.9%), and other psychiatric disorders (22.1%).

Since it is important to examine comorbidity, patients in the CCEP have a coded primary diagnosis and up to six additional diagnoses. For CCEP patients with a primary psychiatric diagnosis, the comorbidity of other diagnoses (second to seventh) are found in Table 3.6.

An examination of only the second diagnosis for comorbidity with a primary psychiatric diagnosis reveals that psychological disorders are the most common at 18.0%, followed by musculoskeletal disorders at 11.1%, ill-defined conditions at 8.2%, digestive diseases at 6.0%, neurological disorders at 4.3%, skin diseases at 3.7%, respiratory diseases at 2.9%, infectious diseases at 1.9%, and neoplasms at 0.6%.

TABLE 3.5 Distribution of Diagnoses for the 4,304 Patients Receiving a Primary Psychiatric Diagnosis

Diagnosis	Percentage	No. of Patients
Mood disorders	34.0	1,461
Somatoform disorders	24.4	1,059
PTSD	14.9	640
Anxiety disorders	5.5	237
Substance abuse	3.5	152
Other diagnoses	17.5	755
Mood disorders can be broken into the following categories:		
Other depressive syndromes	16.0	715
Major depression	8.9	838
Dysthymia	7.4	319
Bipolar disorder	0.7	30
Other mood disorders	0.3	14

TABLE 3.6 Comorbidity of Other Diagnoses for Patients with Primary Psychiatric Diagnosis

Diagnosis	Percentage	No. of Patients
Psychological disorders	40.1	1,735
Neurological disorders	17.1	740
Musculoskeletal disorders	48.4	2,091
Ill-defined conditions	32.9	1,422
Digestive diseases	23.0	995
Skin diseases	17.6	762
Respiratory diseases	13.8	596
Infectious diseases	8.2	356
Neoplasms	2.4	104

4

IOM Review: Difficult-to-Diagnose and Ill-Defined Conditions*

The committee reviewed information on the development of screening instruments in order to contribute to the understanding and assessment of the adequacy of the CCEP protocol. The role of screening in the area of ill-defined conditions is to be able to identify a subset of individuals from a larger group who clearly fit a description of interest. Screening is *not* synonymous with diagnosis. Therefore, the criteria for a good screening instrument are not the same as the criteria for diagnosis.

Screening includes the systematic collection of information. It differs from a survey in that the goal of a survey is to make inferences, whereas the goal of a screening instrument is to identify a particular group of people. It is also important to note that screening does not take place under static conditions. Over time, progress made in the understanding of these conditions will necessitate different generations of the screening instrument. This does not imply that the first instrument developed is bad, but rather that time leads to new knowledge, which leads to the ability to improve the instrument.

A screening instrument should be systematic, quantitative, standardized, and contain tests and procedures which the population to be screened is willing to undergo. The procedures should be specified in advance, one should be able to assign numerical values to nonnumerical characteristics (e.g., the severity of

---

*The material in this section is based, in part, upon presentations and discussion by Dedra S. Buchwald, M.D., Daniel Clauw, M.D., Lt. Col. Tim Cooper, M.D., Nelson Gantz, M.D., Penelope Keyl, M.D., Howard Kipen, M.D., Robert Simms, M.D., and Frederick Wolfe, M.D.

symptoms), and there must be standardized questions and responses. In addition, a good screening instrument does not just ask about the presence or absence of symptoms, it also asks about the presentation of the symptoms; under what circumstances they occur; and their intensity, severity, frequency, and duration (how long before a symptom resolves as well as how long the patient has been experiencing it).

With the development of a good screening instrument, one can elicit important information that will help identify a group of patients about whom one wishes to answer further questions regarding diagnosis and treatment.

CHRONIC FATIGUE SYNDROME

Chronic fatigue syndrome is a clinically defined condition characterized by severe, disabling fatigue that persists for at least 6 months and has a definite onset. The symptoms include self-reported problems in concentration, short-term memory, sleep disturbances, and musculoskeletal pain. A diagnosis is made only after alternative medical and psychiatric causes of fatiguing illness are excluded. There are no diagnostic tests that can validate its diagnosis, no pathognomic medical characteristic that is common to all patients, and no defined treatment that alleviates the symptoms for all patients. A major question surrounding diagnosis of CFS concerns whether CFS or any of its subset is a pathologically discrete entity as opposed to a debilitating but nonspecific condition shared by many different entities.

In 1994, the CDC convened the International Chronic Fatigue Syndrome Study Group to develop a conceptual framework and a set of research guidelines for use in studies of CFS. This group developed the following criteria for defining chronic fatigue syndrome (Fukuda et al., 1994).

A person can be classified as having chronic fatigue syndrome if both of the following criteria are met:

1. clinically evaluated, unexplained, persistent, or relapsing fatigue of new or definite onset that is not due to ongoing exertion, is not substantially relieved by rest, and results in a substantial reduction in previous levels of occupational, educational, social, or personal activities; and

2. the concurrent occurrence of four or more of the following symptoms, all of which must have persisted or recurred for at least six months:

- impaired short-term memory or concentration severe enough to cause substantial reduction in previous levels of activity;
- sore throat;
- tender cervical or axillary lymph nodes;
- muscle pain, multijoint pain without joint swelling or redness;

- headaches of a new type or severity;
- unrefreshing sleep;
- postexertional malaise lasting more than 24 hours.

The minimum laboratory evaluation of patients with suspected CFS includes complete blood count with differential; electrolytes, BUN (blood urea nitrogen), creatinine, calcium, glucose, and thyroid function tests; erythrocyte sedimentation rate; antinuclear antibodies; and urinalysis. Although many patients have significant abnormalities on routine lab tests, uniformity of abnormalities is lacking, and therefore routine laboratory tests cannot be used to determine whether a patient has CFS.

No single cause of CFS has been identified. Of the patients diagnosed with CFS, 80% or more reported that it started with a viral illness. Many suspected agents were reviewed including the Epstein-Barr virus, but none have been found to be causative for CFS. From 60% to 70% of CFS patients reported allergies, compared to 20% of the general population. A variety of tests indicated that there does seem to be heightened reactivity to allergens and a higher prevalence of allergies in patients with chronic fatigue syndrome.

Since allergies are immunologic phenomena, scientists started investigating other potential immunological problems. Findings included decreased natural killer cell number and activity, altered lymphocyte subset numbers and percentage; and increased expression of activation markers on lymphocyte subsets. However, none of these findings was ultimately found to be adequately consistent to be used as a diagnostic measure. Other areas investigated included neuroendocrine and metabolic abnormalities. Although abnormalities do exist in some patients with CFS, there is disagreement over their relevance.

A recent theory is one of dysfunction of the autonomic nervous system. Some of the symptoms of chronic fatigue syndrome can mimic conditions associated with autonomic dysfunction, for example, neurally mediated hypotension. This is a condition in which the general symptoms include light-headedness, sweating, abdominal discomfort, blurred vision, and then presyncope and fainting. The Tilt Table test is used to diagnose neurally mediated hypotension. When Tilt Table testing was applied in a study by Bou-Holaigah et al. (1995), an abnormal response to upright tilt (i.e., development of syncope or severe presyncope with at least a 25 mm Hg decrease in systolic blood pressure and no associated increase in heart rate) was observed in 22 of 23 patients with CFS versus 4 of 14 controls. The authors of the study concluded that CFS is associated with neurally mediated hypotension and that its symptoms may be improved in a subset of patients by therapy directed at this abnormal cardiovascular reflex.

There are conditions that explain the presence of severe fatigue and, therefore, preclude the diagnosis of CFS. These include past or current psychiatric conditions of major depression with melancholic or psychotic features; delusional disorders of any subtype; bipolar affective disorder; schizophrenia of any subtype; dementias of any type; anorexia nervosa; and bulimia.

The following comorbid conditions do not exclude CFS:

- Any condition defined primarily by symptoms that cannot be confirmed by diagnostic laboratory tests (e.g., fibromyalgia, anxiety disorders, somatoform disorders, nonpsychotic or nonmelancholic depression, neurasthenia, panic disorder, and multiple chemical sensitivity disorder).
- Any condition under specific treatment sufficient to alleviate all symptoms related to the condition for which the adequacy of treatment has been well documented (e.g., hypothyroidism in which the adequacy of replacement hormone has been verified by normal thyroid-stimulating hormone levels and asthma in which the adequacy of treatment has been determined by pulmonary function and other testing).
- Any condition that was previously treated with definitive therapy before the development of chronic symptomatic sequelae (e.g., Lyme disease or syphilis).
- Any isolated and unexplained physical examination finding or laboratory or imaging test abnormality that is insufficient to strongly suggest the existence of an exclusionary conditions (e.g., an elevated antinuclear antibody titer that is inadequate to strongly support the diagnosis of a discrete connective tissue disorder without other laboratory or clinical evidence, Fukuda et al., 1994).

The objectives of therapy for CFS are to help the patient develop realistic goals and expectations through education, to provide symptomatic relief, and to preserve and improve the patient's ability to function (Fukuda and Gantz, 1995). A necessary component of this therapy is for the provider to acknowledge that the patient's suffering is real.

Therapy for CFS patients includes provision of symptomatic treatment such as medications for depression, anxiety, pain, sleep problems, and allergies. To prevent further disability it is important for the patient to engage in graded exercise and physical therapy. Cognitive behavioral therapy (CBT) is also used in an attempt to alter attitudes, perceptions, and beliefs that can contribute to maladaptive behavior. Patients need to establish realistic goals for managing their lives, to apply stress reduction techniques, and to restructure their activities to better accommodate their needs and condition. The longer a patient has been ill with CFS, the less likely he or she is to get better. Therefore, early diagnosis and treatment are extremely important.

FIBROMYALGIA

Fibromyalgia (FM) is a disorder of widespread pain, tenderness, fatigue, sleep disturbance, and psychological distress (Wolfe et al., 1995). Additional clinical features may include irritable bowel syndrome, paresthesias, headache, irritable bladder, somatization, and social dysfunction.

Problems with the classification and diagnosis of fibromyalgia led to development of the following criteria by the American College of Rheumatology.

- There must be a history of widespread pain. Pain is considered widespread when all of the following are present:

  — pain in the left side of the body,
  — pain in the right side of the body,
  — pain above the waist, and
  — pain below the waist.

- In addition, axial skeleton pain (cervical spine or anterior chest or thoracic spine or low back) must be present. Shoulder and buttock pain is considered pain for each involved side. "Low back" pain is considered lower segment pain.
- There is pain on digital palpation in 11 of the 18 following sites of tender points:

1. Occiput: bilateral, at the suboccipital muscle insertions.
2. Low cervical: bilateral, at the anterior aspects of the intertransverse spaces at C5–C7.
3. Trapezius: bilateral, at the midpoint of the upper border.
4. Supraspinatus: bilateral, at origins, above the scapular spine near the medial border.
5. Second rib: bilateral, at the second costochondral junctions, just lateral to the junctions on upper surfaces.
6. Lateral epicondyle: bilateral, 2 cm distal to the epicondyles.
7. Gluteal: bilateral, in upper outer quadrants of buttocks in anterior fold of muscle.
8. Greater trochanter: bilateral, posterior to the trochanteric prominence.
9. Knee: bilateral, at the medial fat pad proximal to the joint line.

Fibromyalgia patients can be differentiated from controls by testing their pain threshold or tolerance anywhere on the body, not just on tender points (Clauw, 1995). Fibromyalgia patients have allodynia, a reduction in pain threshold, as well as hyperalgesia, which means that things that hurt are more hurtful. Patients with fibromyalgia may report pain only in certain areas, however, because those areas are the most troublesome. Part of the diagnostic process must, therefore, carefully elicit information about all painful areas. This may be accomplished by using a pain diagram or by asking repeatedly about various body regions.

The major feature distinguishing fibromyalgia from other disorders is tenderness (or sensitivity). The two methods for measuring tenderness are digital palpation and dolorimetry. The amount of force used in palpation is important because too large a force will elicit pain in someone without fibromyalgia, whereas too little force may miss pain in someone with fibromyalgia. It has been suggested that the best method for determining the amount of pressure required is to palpate "normal" individuals of the same build and stature as the suspected fibromyalgia patient. Although questions about the validity of palpation can be raised, studies have shown that trained examiners can reach high levels of agreement in the identification of patients with and without fibromyalgia (Wolfe et al., 1992).

Dolorimetry is a technique that uses a rubber endplate with a spring-loaded force gauge. This gauge is pressed on the tenderpoint site. As the pressure is changed, patients are asked to note when they feel a change from pressure to pain. Although dolorimetry would *appear* to be a more reliable approach than digital palpation to measuring the pain threshold because it eliminates examiner variability in both the amount of pressure used and the interpretation of patient response, data analyses indicate that both digital palpation and manual palpation are more accurate diagnostic approaches. This may be because the gauge is pressed on one site at a time, whereas during palpation, the examiner can feel around for the exact place to exert pressure. In addition, the rolling motion involved in feeling for the correct site may find a tenderness not noted by direct pressure alone (Wolfe, 1994).

In addition to pain, there are other signs and symptoms common to patients with fibromyalgia. In a 1990 ACR study of criteria for the classification of fibromyalgia, 81% of the patients complained of fatigue and 74% complained of sleep disturbance. Psychological factors are also important. Of patients with fibromyalgia, 30% report the symptom of depression (Wolfe, 1994). It is important to point out that fibromyalgia cannot be explained solely as a psychiatric illness like depression, however.

Family members of fibromyalgia patients have a higher-than-expected rate of fibromyalgia. In addition, trauma, either physical or emotional, may precipitate one-third of the cases of fibromyalgia. Infections such as Lyme disease and HIV and connective tissue disorders such as systemic lupus erythematosus and rheumatoid arthritis frequently coexist with fibromyalgia. Aerobic fitness may be a positive modulating factor, that is, it may lessen the negative effects of the condition (Clauw, 1995).

Many investigators now agree that aberrant central nervous system mechanisms are likely to be responsible for the majority of clinical findings in fibromyalgia. A central nervous system genesis explains not only the high incidence of nonmusculoskeletal symptoms in a wide variety of organs and tissues, but also the affective disorders and neurological features which occur in this condition (Clauw, 1995).

Available treatments for fibromyalgia range from conventional medication therapy with tricyclic antidepressants to nonconventional interventions such as biofeedback. It appears that there is short-term benefit in the treatment of fibromyalgia syndrome with tricyclic agents, but this has not proved long-lasting in placebo-controlled trials. A relatively small proportion of patients (about 25% to 30%) have significant improvement. The majority have little or no improvement.

In addition to commonly used pharmacologic therapies, patient education, reassurance, and an exercise program can each play an important role in relieving the symptoms associated with this musculoskeletal syndrome. Patient education is important in assuring patients that they have a common, nonthreatening condition. Such education should include a description of how the diagnosis was made, what the condition represents, and the entire therapeutic plan. In addition to education, exercise has been shown to contribute to improvement in pain threshold scores.

Electromyography (EMG) biofeedback has been tested in controlled trial settings. Ferraccioli et al. (1987) conducted a controlled study of biofeedback in 12 patients and reported a 50% clinical improvement in 9 of those patients, sustained for six months. A study of electroacupuncture showed improvement in the active treatment group, but limitations to the study include no measure of functional or psychological status, lack of specification of time of follow-up assessment, the fact that patients may not have been optimally blinded, and no determination of whether electroacupuncture is equivalent to acupuncture.

It appears that whereas the most effective short-term treatment for fibromyalgia is antidepressant therapy, the long-term efficacy of treatment remains elusive.

MULTIPLE CHEMICAL SENSITIVITY

Multiple chemical sensitivity (MCS) is a diagnosis given to patients who, in response to a chemical exposure that is tolerated by most individuals, exhibit a variety of symptoms that have no apparent organic (or physiologic) basis. MCS is reported to result from a single episode or recurring episodes of a chemical exposure, such as solvent or pesticide poisoning, but it also arises without reports of untoward initial exposure. There is very little agreement on what the symptoms represent, and no definition has yet been endorsed for clinical use by a body of physicians. The American Medical Association (AMA) and the American College of Physicians have both considered the general topic but have not yet recognized a specific disease entity or definition.

Cullen's definition of MCS, primarily for research purposes, appears to be the most widely accepted. The definition allows physicians to distinguish MCS from other clusters of commonly experienced symptoms (Sparks et al., 1994a. This definition has four characteristics:

1. MCS is *acquired* in relation to some documentable environmental exposure that may initially have produced a demonstrable toxic effect. This aspect excludes patients with long-standing health problems who later attribute certain symptoms to chemical exposure.
2. Symptoms involve more than one organ system, and they recur and abate in response to *predictable* environmental stimuli.
3. Symptoms are elicited by exposures to chemicals that are demonstrable but very low (perhaps several standard deviations below the average exposures known to cause toxic or irritant health effects in humans).
4. The manifestations of MCS are *subjective.* No widely available test of organ system function can explain the symptoms, and there is no objective evidence of organ system damage or dysfunction. The syndrome may be severely distressing and functionally disabling, however, because patients increasingly attempt to avoid chemical exposures.

The chemicals most closely associated with the majority of initiating episodes are organic solvents, pesticides, and respiratory irritants. This could be because of the widespread use of these materials. The other common setting in which many cases are reported is in buildings with indoor air problems (Cullen, 1997).

There are many theories of the etiology of multiple chemical sensitivity. One perspective has focused on the relationship between the mucosae of the upper respiratory tract and the limbic system, especially the linkage in the nose. MCS patients typically report heightened odor sensitivity. Findings suggest that MCS patients do not detect odors at lower thresholds than others, but they may respond more markedly once odors are detected. The relationship of this finding to reports of inflammatory nasal pathology and increased nasal resistance is unexplored, but the pathologic findings require confirmation with controlled studies.

Others have suggested that MCS might be related to a disturbance of the immune system. No controlled and blinded studies have been published demonstrating a consistent pattern of alteration in immune parameters in MCS patients after chemical exposure (Sparks et al., 1994a). Another hypothesis is that chemical exposures produce toxic free radicals that cause cell membranes to release inflammatory mediators. No scientific data have been put forth to support this theory, however (Sparks et al., 1994a).

Another theory is that psychological mechanisms explain MCS. It has been proposed that MCS may be a manifestation of the human response to stress or a conditioned response to an initial toxic experience (Jewett, 1992). Some have hypothesized that MCS is a late-life response to early childhood traumas such as sexual abuse. Some investigators argue that MCS is a misdiagnosed psychiatric disease such as depression, anxiety disorders, somatization disorders, or other common psychiatric disorders (Sparks et al., 1994a).

Many scientists, physicians, and others have postulated that MCS is, in many ways, a belief system promoted by clinical ecologists and those sympathetic to their views and followed by medically unsophisticated persons. As part of this scenario, MCS patients view themselves as victims of external and uncontrollable factors, and they reject the concept that symptoms are not indicative of severe disease and may have psychological components. A factor that may contribute to this belief system is the increasing concern of the public regarding environmental pollution and the health effects of exposure to man-made chemicals (Sparks et al., 1994a).

Although a great deal of literature can be found on the pathogenesis of MCS, there is little clinical or experimental evidence that supports strongly any of the views put forth. The available evidence shows that patients diagnosed with MCS are very heterogeneous and that particular health belief models, concurrent psychiatric illness, and psychologic stress characterize a vulnerable group of people who then develop a sensitivity to odors or low-level chemical irritants (Sparks et al., 1994b). Despite the lack of agreement on etiology, clinicians can still help affected patients with their symptoms.

There are no laboratory findings that are characteristic of MCS. To consider this diagnosis, one must take a history and elicit both the symptoms and the fact that they wax and wane with exposure to real agents that are tolerated by most people. Diagnostic testing is done primarily to rule out other illness in the differential diagnosis. Diagnostic evaluation of the suspected MCS patient includes the following:

A. History
- Detailed exposure history (workplace and other environmental exposures)
- Industrial hygiene data (Material Safety Data Sheets, results of exposure monitoring, etc.)
- Current and past medical illnesses and results of previous diagnostic work-ups and treatments
- Review of prior medical records

B. Physical examination to rule out other illnesses in the differential diagnosis

C. Consultation
- Occupational and environmental medicine specialist
- Psychiatrist
- Other specialists as appropriate to rule out other medical conditions in the differential diagnosis

D. Other
- Symptom diary (this *can* cause people to be overly focused on things they might otherwise ignore)
- Short-term removal from exposure

The focus of treatment is to acknowledge that the symptoms are real and distressing even if there is no evidence of observable organic pathology. The goal of therapy is the control of symptoms. Success depends on the patient's improved understanding of the role stress plays in exacerbating symptoms and on the acquisition of skills for coping with the impact of the illness on daily life (Sparks et al., 1994b). Treatment should be individualized but should include enhancing the patient's sense of control over workplace or home stressors. Approaches to reducing stress have included massage, physical therapy, meditation, or regular exercise. The patient should be reassured that MCS is not fatal and is not associated with signs of progressive disease.

A recommendation for complete avoidance of chemical exposures is not indicated because there is no evidence for a cumulative toxic injury and it is impossible to accomplish. Treatment could also include medication to control symptoms, an increase in physical and social activity, and treatment of other coexisting medical illnesses. It is very important to treat coexisting psychiatric manifestations such as depression and panic attacks. Such treatments may be helpful in controlling symptoms no matter what the etiology.

CONTROVERSIES AND OVERLAP

Patients with CFS, fibromyalgia, and MCS have many symptoms in common. According to some investigations, these conditions may represent overlapping clinical syndromes. In a study by Buchwald and Garrity (1994), it was found that 70% of patients with fibromyalgia and 30% of those with MCS met the criteria for CFS. A study by Hudson et al. found that 42% of fibromyalgia patients have met the criteria for CFS (1992), and research conducted by Wysenbeek et al. (1991) found that 21% of FM patients met CFS criteria. Goldenberg et al. (1990) found that 70% of patients diagnosed as having CFS met the ACR criteria for fibromyalgia.

There are other disorders that overlap with CFS. For patients with TMD, or temporomandibular disorder (also known as TMJ arthritis), almost 60% have the CFS symptom of fatigue for more than six months (Buchwald and Garrity, et al., 1994) and 30% meet the second part of the definition, which is reduced activity. Another overlapping syndrome on which little has been published is Sjögren's syndrome, an autoimmune disorder. One study (Calabrese et al., 1994) produced results that seemed to indicate there was a subset of CFS patients who have a Sjögren's-like syndrome, with dry eyes, dry mouth, and at least some of the laboratory abnormalities seen in Sjögren's syndrome.

The cardinal features of these illnesses are chronic regional or chronic widespread pain in the absence of nociceptive input, fatigue, and dysfunction of visceral organs or sensory amplification. Individuals who have multiple chemical sensitivity, for example, sometimes find that they are sensitive to many kinds of sensory input such as bright lights and loud noises. Therefore, if one defines a group of individuals in the population that has a high degree of pain or that has a high degree of fatigue or any of these symptoms, many of the individuals will also have a number of other symptoms. However, it is difficult to define the degree of pain or to rate the pain as to intensity.

Fatigue is likewise a problem. Accurate tools to quantify fatigue have yet to be developed and accepted. Therefore it is difficult to define a pathological degree of fatigue. Anywhere one decides to draw the line results in an arbitrary distinction. The minor symptoms (headaches, constipation, etc.) are also problematic. A number of population-based studies have shown that the more of these symptoms individuals have, the more likely they are to have psychological or psychiatric comorbidities.

Whatever diagnostic label is arrived at, patients in this spectrum of illness will have a higher than normal incidence of things such as tension and migraine headaches, affective disorders, TMD, irritable bowel syndrome, and so on. Fibromyalgia is a diagnosis which defines an extreme of pain and tenderness experienced by 3% to 4% of the general population. CFS defines a smaller percentage of the population that is most fatigued. In reality, fatigue and pain or tenderness in the population occur on a continuum. What is seen for all of these different symptoms is that they occur over a wide continuum in the population and that current definitions attempt to draw a line somewhere and say that one side of the line represents illness and the other, wellness.

5

IOM Review: Stress, Psychiatric Disorders, and Their Relationship to Physical Signs and Symptoms*

In May 1997, the committee convened a workshop of research and clinical experts in the areas of stress (including military stress), the effects of stress on the endocrine and immune systems, substance abuse, posttraumatic stress disorder (PTSD), depression, and subthreshold depression. Presentations were focused on providing the latest information in these areas that could assist the committee in its review of the adequacy of the Comprehensive Clinical Evaluation Program in diagnosing stress and psychiatric disorders and in determining whether or not effective treatments existed for these conditions.

STRESSORS AND STRESS

As discussed earlier, individuals deployed to the Persian Gulf were exposed to a number of stressors. The term stressors generally refers to the external circumstances that challenge or obstruct an individual. Stress, on the other hand, is the state of arousal resulting from the presence of socioenvironmental demands that tax the ordinary adaptive capacity of the individual. Production of stress is an environment person interaction and is influenced by such characteristics as needs, values, perceived ability to respond, and coping skills.

---

*The material in this section is based, in part, on presentations by Hagop Akiskal, M.D., Carol Aneshensel, Ph.D., Firdaus Dhabhar, Ph.D., MAJ Charles Engel, M.D., David Foy, Ph.D., Walter Ling, M.D., MAJ Michael Roy, M.D., and John D. Wynn, M.D.

There are two broad types of stressors: (1) eventful changes that have a discrete onset and a discrete cessation and (2) chronic stressors that emerge from ongoing situations until it becomes apparent that there is a problem. Most chronic stressors are related to the ongoing nature of social organization and social roles. Other chronic stressors include daily hassles (e.g., a slowdown on the freeway) and ambient stressors (e.g., deteriorating aspects of a neighborhood).

Life event stressors refer to objective changes in life circumstances that are of sufficient magnitude to change a person's usual activities (e.g., acute physical illness). These can be expected to occur throughout the life course, and it is the undesirable events that are stressful for people.

Stress proliferation refers to the notion that a particular stressful circumstance is usually not confined in a person's life but tends to spread out and create additional problems in other areas of life (i.e., a primary stressor may produce a secondary stressor). Primary stressors are primary in the sense that they are the root origin of a series of other problematic life circumstances called secondary stressors. These secondary stressors are not necessarily secondary in their potency and refer to the spillover of the primary stressor into other aspects of a person's life (e.g., interference with job, disruption of relationships with family and friends, constriction of social activities).

For traumatic events, if secondary adversities or other stressors arise, the effects may be additive, that is, they may proliferate.

Once these additional or secondary stressors have been created, they then serve as an independent source of stress. Stress may proliferate for the individual who is the primary target of interest and also for the family and friends of that individual.

In general, the duration of an exposure is related to the effects of stress. The more long term the exposure, the more long term are the effects. In addition, just because a person is removed from a stressful life circumstance, the effects of having been in that condition or circumstance persist, even though the stressor is absent.

The Gulf War had many very stressful experiences, despite the fact that it was a military success. There were many months leading up to the war in which the US troops were uncertain about the strength of Iraqi troops, whether chemical or biological weapons would be used, and whether they would be injured or killed in the engagement. In addition, troops were rapidly and unexpectedly deployed, separated from family and friends, faced with a harsh desert environment and environmental hazards, and exposed to a direct life threat; they also witnessed death and destruction.

When individuals deployed to the Gulf returned home, it was assumed that since the war itself was brief and the level of loss of US lives was low, problems associated with the war would be few. The Department of Veterans Affairs did develop a Persian Gulf Registry as a means of addressing questions about possible future effects of air pollutant exposure and other environmental agents, particularly those associated with the oil well fires. However, as time passed, it became apparent that there were concerns about a number of exposure issues.

Information on exposures and their health consequences was contradictory and, as such, potentially worsened the already stressful situation by making it ambiguous. Because the perception that one has something wrong with one's body is itself a source of stress, the very vagueness surrounding the information that was forthcoming about agents to which one was exposed and the lack of knowledge of health consequences of such exposures have exacerbated the impact of the stress associated with health complaints.

In determining the negative effects created by exposure to stress, it is necessary to look beyond the one primary stressor to the creation of problems in other areas of a person's life and, additionally, in the lives of people with whom he or she is in close association.

CONSEQUENCES OF STRESS

Research has shown that stressors have been associated with major depression, symptoms of depression and anxiety, alcohol abuse and dependence, and substance abuse and dependence. Many of these conditions are undiagnosed in primary care populations for a number of reasons including the training and experience of the examiner, the time pressure for completing examinations, stigmatization and social attitudes, and the misperception that treatment does not work.

Depression

The diagnosis of depression in the primary care setting is frequently missed, and when properly diagnosed, depression is often inadequately treated. A 4-year longitudinal study of medical outcomes was begun in the late 1980s and involved more than 20,000 patients in three centers (Boston, Los Angeles, and Chicago) and different financing systems. General medical clinicians saw 364 patients and were aware that the focus of the study was depression. Despite this fact, these primary care physicians missed the diagnosis of depression 50% of the time (Wells and Burnham, 1991).

Of the patients found by screening during the primary care visit to have a major ongoing depression, 59% received no medication and were not in psychotherapy. Of those who received medication, 19% received only a minor tranquilizer, and 12% only an antidepressant, and of the ones receiving antidepressants, 39% received homeopathic doses. The underdiagnosis, then, was compounded by undertreatment.

To facilitate the task of diagnosing mental disorders, primary care providers must become familiar with diagnostic categories, historical features, and interview techniques.

There are three diagnostic categories of major mental disorders: (1) mood disorders, (2) anxiety disorders, and (3) psychotic disorders. A mood disorder is a diagnosis established on the basis of a recurrent pattern of mood episodes. Mood episodes are a group of signs and symptoms that co-occur for a minimal duration of time. They can be part of a mood disorder, a psychotic disorder, or a general medical disorder. Kinds of mood episodes include major depressive, manic, mixed, and hypomanic.

To identify a major depressive episode, one looks for either a persistent depressed mood that occurs every day or most of the day and lasts at least two weeks, *or* diminished interest or pleasure in all or almost all activities *and* five of the following: significant weight loss or change in appetite; insomnia or hypersomnia nearly every day; psychomotor retardation or agitation (observable); fatigue or loss of energy; feelings of worthlessness or excessive (or inappropriate) guilt; diminished ability to think, concentrate, or make decisions; recurrent thoughts of death or suicide, or a suicide attempt.

A manic episode includes a distinct period of abnormally and persistently elevated, expansive, or irritable mood necessitating hospitalization or lasting at least one week *and* three or more of the following: inflated self-esteem or grandiosity; decreased need for sleep; greater talkativeness than usual or pressure to keep talking; flight of ideas or racing thoughts; distractibility; or risky measurable activities or endangerment.

There are different kinds of mania. The dysphoric or mixed episode is a combination of mania and depression, characterized by marked impairment. The hypomanic episode is not severe enough to show impairment in social or occupational functioning or to necessitate hospitalization, and there are no psychotic features.

The language of episodes can be translated into the language of the primary care clinician. An episode is a syndrome (i.e., a collection of signs and symptoms). Syndromes lead to clinical evaluation; to differential diagnosis, and ultimately, to clinical diagnosis, prognosis, and treatment. Disorders are diagnoses.

Mood disorders are divided into depressive disorders and bipolar disorders. The depressive disorders include major depression (one or more major depressive episodes), minor depression (sadness and/or anhedonia, at least one more symptom of major depression, and two weeks impairment and/or distress), and dysthymia (2 years or more of a depressed mood for "more days than not," two or more neurovegetative symptoms, and has never met criteria for major depressive episode).

Depression is further divided into melancholic, chronic, and other types. Melancholic depressions often do not respond well to treatment, and result in decreasing activity and marked sleep disturbances with a worse prognosis. The chronic type of depression lasts at least 2 years in a row without any remission of more than 2 months, and later intervention results in slower recovery. This is not dysthmia.

Misdiagnosis is often to due to the fact that there is an overlap in the signs and symptoms of depression with many medical conditions. A common error begins with the idea, "Well wouldn't you be depressed if you were so sick?" In addition, the clinical presentation of depression includes confusing or ambiguous (non-mood) complaints such as pervasive boredom, decreased energy, insomnia, and fatigue. Another presentation is irritability. Patients may say they feel sad all the time—or depressed, hopeless, pessimistic, or blue. There are some patients who seek care because they have vague or nonspecific physical complaints such as fatigue, loss of energy, sleep difficulties, or unexplained somatic symptoms.

A number of instruments can be used to screen for depression. These include the Beck Depression Inventory, the Zung Self-rating Depression Scale (SDS), the Center for Epidemiological Studies-Depression Scale (CES-D), and the Inventory to Diagnose Depression (IDD). When in doubt about a diagnosis of any mental disorder, a physician should schedule early follow-up to confirm or deny the diagnosis and to let the patient know that the physician is concerned. It has been shown that as many as 15% of patients with inadequately treated depression kill themselves.

In diagnosing depression in primary care, it is important to screen populations at elevated risk, to increase the clinical sensitivity of primary care providers, to ensure that there is adequate time to perform the evaluation, to remove barriers to specialty care, to encourage multidisciplinary management, to assess comorbidity, and to overcome stereotypes.

Posttraumatic Stress Disorder

Posttraumatic stress disorder (PTSD) appeared as an official diagnosis in the American Psychiatric Association's 1980 publication of the *Diagnostic and Statistical Manual of Mental Disorders* (*DSM-III*). PTSD was recognized as a new disorder, linked to external stressors that are overwhelming and extreme. PTSD has been found to be frequent in veterans of military combat and represents an important concern in providing care to the veteran population. In the National Vietnam Veterans Readjustment Study, investigators found that an estimated 15.2% of all male Vietnam War theater veterans (about 479,000 American men) met the criteria for current PTSD at the time the data were compiled (Rundell and Ursano, 1996). A study by Southwick et al. (1995) found that in a 2-year follow-up to a study of Persian Gulf veterans conducted 6 months after the war's end, "although symptoms were relatively mild, there was an overall increase in PTSD symptoms at 2 years, and not before." They go on to suggest that it may take time for the consequences of traumatic exposure to become apparent.

The required features of PTSD are a traumatic event that precipitates symptoms of a crisis reaction in the individual (i.e., the individual was overwhelmed physiologically and showed signs of extreme horror, helplessness, or grief, in the case of a tragic loss). This is frequently referred to as Criterion A. Other required features are that the trauma be reexperienced in dreams or thoughts or that it be reenacted, that there be a numbing of responsiveness, and that at least two of the following symptoms occur: hyperalertness (exaggerated startle response), sleep disturbance, guilt, trouble concentrating, avoidance of activities prompting recall of the original event, and worsening of symptoms by exposure to events resembling the original event (Helzer et al., 1987).

For providers not experienced in the diagnosis of PTSD, the most common error is to make the assumption that the only requirement for satisfying Criterion A is to determine whether the individual personally experienced a traumatic event (e.g., served in a hostile fire zone). However, the provider must go beyond this to elicit the individual's response to the trauma (i.e., the extent to which he or she experienced reactions such as intense fear, helplessness, and horror).

Although direct exposure is probably the most potent, observational experiences (e.g., observing horrific things happening to others) cannot be disregarded as traumatic events. Vicarious exposure, especially in the case of close social distance to the victim, is also capable of producing PTSD symptoms.

It has been well documented from both clinical and epidemiological data that combat-related PTSD is frequently associated with other psychiatric morbidity, and it has been suggested that alcohol and substance use have a role in precipitating anxiety and mood-related symptoms (Mellman et al., 1992). In addition, individuals with PTSD are at risk for developing secondary affective, alcohol and substance abuse, as well as panic and phobic disorders. Treatment of these comorbid conditions is essential to the management of PTSD (Marmar et al., 1993). According to Marmar et al., the severity and course of PTSD are influenced by the interaction of the traumatic stress exposure with a background of individual psychological and biological vulnerability.

Substance Abuse

Substance abuse problems are fairly prevalent in primary care. About 20% to 30% of patients who visit primary care physicians do so for problems that relate in some way to substance abuse or misuse. Substance abuse results from addiction, which is a disease process characterized by the compulsive use of a specific psychoactive substance. An individual engages in a set of behaviors regarding the substance that can lead to a dependence disorder or an abuse disorder.

In terms of substance abuse, the role of the primary care physician is twofold. First, the primary care physician must assess and treat the medical problems related to substance abuse. There are, for example, a number of medical diseases related to parenteral drug use such as endocarditis, acute hepatitis, cirrhosis, bleeding ulcers, pancreatitis, stroke, seizures, amnesia, dementia, and certain cardiovascular and pulmonary diseases, as well as overdose, trauma, and hormonal abnormalities. Medical problems that result from alcohol abuse include neurological problems, liver disease, pancreatic disease, and hematologic diseases. There is also a great deal of comorbidity between substance abuse and psychiatric disorders such as schizophrenia, affective disorders, anxiety disorders, and antisocial personality disorders.

The second major responsibility of the primary care physician is to conduct substance abuse screening. If a patient presents with a medical problem related to substance abuse, the primary care physician should screen for abuse as a cause of the problem. A very important component of this screening is to determine the severity of the problem and the risk of complications. To conduct effective screening, the physician must interview the patient concerning his or her general health habits, diet and exercise, use of prescriptions, use of over-the-counter and home remedies, smoking, drinking, and use of marijuana and other drugs. In addition, the primary care physician should use one of the substance abuse screening instruments (e.g., CAGE, MAST/DAST, AUDIT, HSS, and the T-ACE/TWEAK; see Appendix I for copies of the instruments).

Other Consequences

Stress has also been associated with various physical health problems, particularly immune system functioning. A study by Cohen et al. (1991) showed that for individuals inoculated with a cold virus (rhinovirus type 2, 9, or 14, respiratory syncytial viruses, or coronavirus type 229E), there was an increased infection rate in those who reported a high level of recent stress. According to work conducted recently at Rockefeller University, it appears that moderate stress (i.e., stress that is circumscribed both in its physical duration and its perception), maintained in a healthy individual, seems to enhance cell-mediated immunity. There is also evidence that it might enhance humoral or antibody-dependent immunity. However, chronic stress disrupts equilibrium and decreases cell-mediated immunity (Dhabhar presentation, 1997).

There are other potential consequences of stress for health outcomes, for example, the effects of stress on health behavior. Some behaviors may produce positive effects (e.g., running as a coping mechanism), whereas many are unhealthy (e.g., smoking, drinking, overeating). Stress exerts an indirect effect on health via these kinds of behaviors.

There are also stress effects on illness behavior, that is, what a person does who perceives him or herself as having some sort of sickness. It has been accepted for many years that persons who engage in certain types of stressful behavior are at higher risk of developing coronary heart disease (Williams, 1995). Less well known is the fact that those who suffer from clinical depression experience a 5-fold higher mortality following myocardial infarction than nondepressed patients.

According to Chrousos and Gold (1992), a stress system within the body produces pathophysiologic states that can make a person vulnerable to a range of disorders, including endocrine, inflammatory, and psychiatric disorders. It has also been shown that jobs that place high demands on a worker while allowing little latitude in deciding how the demands are met create high job strain. Employment in high-strain jobs has been associated with increased ambulatory blood pressure levels (Schnall et al., 1992).

Friedman and Schnurr (1995) conducted a review of the literature on physical health outcomes associated with traumatic events including exposure to a war zone, sexual or other criminal victimization, natural or human-made disasters, and serious accidents. They concluded that "the trauma and health literature is impressive for the consistency of results showing that exposure to catastrophic stress is associated with adverse health reports, medical utilization, morbidity, and mortality among survivors." Although there is some concern that this literature includes work with methodological flaws, Friedman and Schnurr (1995) emphasized that there was "general consistency of findings across diverse trauma populations and outcomes . . .," including morbidity and mortality data that supported self-report and utilization data.

6

Conclusions and Recommendations

A great deal of time and effort has been expended evaluating DoD's Comprehensive Clinical Evaluation Program. It has been reviewed by the President's Advisory Committee, the General Accounting Office, the Office of Technology Assessment, the Institute of Medicine, and many other organizations. As more is learned, it becomes easier to focus on the kinds of questions the CCEP should be asking. As Dr. Penelope Keyl said in her workshop presentation on the development of good screening instruments, progress made over time will necessitate new generations of screening instruments. This does not imply that the first instrument developed is bad, but rather that time leads to new knowledge, which leads to the ability to improve the instrument.

Such is the case with the CCEP. Over time, the CCEP and other programs have generated information that has led us to focus on areas of importance for those concerned about the health consequences of Persian Gulf deployment. This information has enabled us to take a closer look, to make a more thorough examination of the system, and to identify areas in which change will be of benefit. The committee believes that such change is healthy, that it reflects growth, and that it should be a natural part of any system having as one of its goals the delivery of high-quality health care services.

Change also occurs with individuals. It may be that as time passes or new information is released, some of those who have already participated in the CCEP will develop new concerns or problems. The committee hopes that DoD will encourage these individuals to return to the CCEP for further evaluation and diagnosis.

The committee wishes to emphasize that it is impressed with the dedication and concern exhibited by DoD personnel with whom committee members met. These individuals are knowledgeable regarding Persian Gulf issues and willing to learn more about identifying and resolving areas of concern for improving the health of active-duty personnel deployed to the Gulf.

MEDICALLY UNEXPLAINED SYMPTOM SYNDROMES

The committee spent some time deliberating on the precise meaning of "difficult to diagnose" or "ill defined" as a description of a category of conditions. When labeling something as difficult to diagnose, one usually means that special expertise is required to arrive at a diagnosis, but many of these conditions do not require such expertise. Chronic fatigue syndrome, fibromyalgia, and multiple chemical sensitivity are symptom complexes that have a great deal of overlap in the symptoms present in each condition but are well defined clinically, even if they are medically unexplained. Despite the fact that they are medically unexplained, they may cause significant impairment and they are illnesses that are only understood through time, that is, it requires the passage of time and the evaluation of responses to treatment to arrive at these diagnoses. The committee decided, therefore, to refer to this spectrum of illnesses as *medically unexplained symptom syndromes.* This spectrum of illnesses may include those which are etiologically unexplained, lack currently detectable pathophysiological changes, and/or cannot currently be diagnostically labeled.

These medically unexplained symptom syndromes are often associated with depression and anxiety. There remains a debate about how to distinguish these syndromes from psychiatric diagnoses, but it is clear that they are not simply psychiatric diagnoses. However, since most of the recommended treatments for medically unexplained symptom syndromes overlap with the pharmacological and behavioral treatments for psychological conditions or psychiatric diagnoses, the committee believes that it is important to identify and evaluate the symptoms associated with these conditions and then treat those symptoms.

The committee recommends that when patients presenting with medically unexplained symptom syndromes are evaluated, the provider must have access to the full and complete medical record, including previous use of services. The presence of such information is important because adequate evaluation of these disorders involves a longitudinal perspective that includes response to treatment.

In the area of medically unexplained symptom syndromes, it is sometimes not possible to arrive at a definitive diagnosis. It may be possible, however, to treat the presenting complaints or symptoms. **The committee recommends that in cases where a diagnosis cannot be identified, treatment should be**

targeted to specific symptoms or syndromes (e.g., fatigue, pain, depression). If these symptoms and conditions are left untreated, they can become chronic and potentially disabling. **The committee recommends that the CCEP be encouraged to identify patients in this spectrum of illnesses early in the process of their disease. In addition, primary care providers should identify the patients' functional impairments so as to be able to suggest treatments that will help improve these disabilities.**

STRESS

In this group of medically unexplained symptom syndromes it is important to recognize and acknowledge that the problems and stress facing the patient will continue to be difficult. Stress is a major issue in the lives of patients within this spectrum of illness. Stress need not be looked at so much as a causative agent, but rather as a part of the condition of the patient that cannot be ignored. With these medically unexplained symptom syndromes, the potential for stress proliferation is great among both the person deployed to the Persian Gulf and the family members.

Media attention and reports by the military to Gulf War veterans that toxic exposure could have occurred are very stressful events, regardless of anyone's efforts to explain what happened. Such announcements carry with them stressful burdens for the veteran. The stress associated with these reports of and worry over toxic exposures needs to be recognized and addressed.

Research has shown that stressors have been associated with major depression, substance abuse, and various physical health problems. Those deployed to the Gulf were exposed to a vast array of different stressors that carry with them their own potential health consequences. Current collection of exposure information does not adequately address an investigation of traumatic events to which the deployed soldier may have been exposed. **The committee recommends that the CCEP contain questions on traumatic event exposures in addition to the exposure information currently being collected. This would include the addition of open-ended questions that ask the patient to list the events that were most upsetting to him or her while deployed. Positive responses to questions regarding such events, as well as to other exposure questions, should be pursued with a *narrative inquiry*, which would address such items as the specific nature of the exposure; the duration; the frequency of repetition; the dose or intensity (if appropriate); whether the patient was taking protective measures and, if so, what these measures were; and the symptoms manifested.**

Other suggestions for questions that could be added to the CCEP include the following: When did you first have questions or worries about being exposed? When did you first hear other information on possible exposures?

What were your responses to that information? Providers in the CCEP need to take a history that includes some narrative to allow the veteran to express how he or she feels.

It is always important to understand and acknowledge that the patients' complaints are real. It is certainly important for providers in the CCEP to do so when attempting to identify and address the health concerns of Persian Gulf veterans. Furthermore, no matter what additional information may be forthcoming about potential exposures to toxins and their effects, **the committee recommends that DoD providers acknowledge stressors as a legitimate but not necessarily sole cause of physical symptoms and conditions.**

The committee believes that there are certain jobs undertaken in the midst of war that, by their very nature, result in high stress (e.g. grave registration duty). The effect of stress associated with these jobs can be mitigated if approached properly. **The committee recommends that the DoD provide special training and debriefing for those who are engaged in high-risk jobs such as those associated with the Persian Gulf experience.** Every soldier who goes to war will be subjected to major disturbing events since war by its very nature involves death and destruction. **The committee recommends that DoD provide to each about-to-be deployed soldier risk or hazard communication which is well developed and designed to provide information regarding what the individual can expect and the potentially traumatic events to which he or she might be exposed.**

The committee wishes to emphasize that the accurate diagnosis of patients with medically unexplained symptom syndromes and/or conditions induced or exacerbated by upsetting events requires the expenditure of time, time in which the provider and the patient interact. It is not possible to hand the patient a questionnaire and expect that all necessary information will be revealed. In a world of time constraints and tightly scheduled appointments, **the committee recommends that adequate time must be provided during initial interactions with patients in the CCEP in order to ensure that all pertinent information is forthcoming.** The committee believes that the patient-physician interaction should be fostered, and the perception that evaluation is directed by the clock should be avoided.

SCREENING

Depression is a condition that is common in primary care. Most individuals who experience depression continue to function, but if they are left untreated, their condition deteriorates. Unlike many of the medically unexplained symptom syndromes, there are effective treatments for depression. The data presented indicate rising rates of depression among those examined in the CCEP but no evidence that individuals are being properly diagnosed or treated according to currently accepted clinical practice guidelines. There are many self-rated screening tests (e.g., the Beck Depression Inventory [BDI], the Zung Scale, the Center for Epidemiological Studies-Depression Scale [CES-D], the Inventory to Diagnose Depression [IDD]) that could be used as a first-level screen at the primary care level.

The committee recommends that there be increased screening at the primary care level for depression. Every primary care physician should have a simple standardized screen for depression. If a patient scores in the significant range, this person should be referred to a qualified mental health professional for further evaluation and treatment. If depression is identified, there has to be more questioning on exposure to traumatic problems.

There has been a great deal of concern evinced about the possibility of widespread PSTD in those deployed to the Persian Gulf. Most of the individuals identified as having PTSD are diagnosed following a structured interview at Phase II. However, the committee believes that there are those who have *some* of the symptoms of PTSD or of depression but are not true PTSD cases yet might be helped with treatment of their symptoms.

The committee recommends that any individual who reports any significant PTSD symptoms and/or a significant traumatic stressor should be referred to a qualified mental health professional for further evaluation and treatment.

Substance abuse or misuse problems are prevalent in primary care. In addition, individuals with untreated depression or with medically unexplained symptom syndromes may have an enhanced risk of substance abuse. (See Appendix I for examples of screening instruments.) **The committee recommends, therefore, that every primary care physician should have a simple, standardized screen for substance abuse. Every individual who screens positive should be referred for further treatment and evaluation.**

There are certain areas in which baseline assessments are of immense value in the clinical evaluation of an individual patient's status (e.g., pulmonary function and neurobehavioral testing). Changes in neurocognitive and peripheral nerve function are measured by comparing the individual's current status to a baseline measure. This is also true for measuring complaints of memory impairment. Individual baseline information is necessary because the variability across individuals is too great to identify a generalized "normal" screening level.

The committee recommends that DoD explore the possibility of using neurobehavioral testing at entry into the military to determine whether it is feasible to use such tests to predict change in functioning or track change in function during a soldier's military career.

PROGRAM EVALUATION

Most patients in the CCEP receive a diagnosis after completing a Phase I examination; some are referred to Phase II for evaluation; and a few have gone on to participate in the program at the Specialized Care Center. Information presented to the committee indicates that there is great variation across regions in the percentage of patients who are diagnosed as having primary psychiatric diagnoses. A determination of the reasons for this variation should be made. Although there may be many reasons, one explanation could relate to the consistency with which procedures for diagnosis and referral are implemented from facility to facility. **The committee recommends that an evaluation be conducted to examine (1) the consistency with which Phase I examinations are conducted across facilities; (2) the patterns of referral from Phase I to Phase II; and (3) the adequacy of treatment provided to certain categories of patients where there is the potential for great impact on patient outcomes when effective treatment is rendered (e.g., depression).**

This effort could be facilitated by the development and use of clinical practice guidelines such as those currently being developed by the Department of Veterans Affairs and many medical specialties. Clinical practice guidelines are systematically developed statements that assist practitioners and patients in decision making about appropriate health care for specific clinical circumstances (IOM, 1992). The process of developing these guidelines could also serve as an opportunity for increased learning for providers since their participation is crucial to successful implementation.

The Specialized Care Center at Walter Reed Army Medical Center has provided evaluation and treatment to 78 patients. A great deal of effort and thought has gone into the development of a program designed to help the patient understand his or her conditions and engage in behaviors most likely to result in improvement. The committee was asked to assess the effectiveness of this center within the context of medically unexplained symptom syndromes, stress, and psychiatric disorders. As the committee began its discussion of the effectiveness of the Specialized Care Center it became apparent that such an assessment was dependent on a number of factors that have not been well defined. What is the goal of the center—is it treatment, research, or education? Should a major consideration in the center's evaluation be the cost of services? Should the numbers of those receiving care be taken into consideration, and if so, what are the barriers to patients accessing this level of care?

The committee concluded that at this time, it is not possible to conduct a fair or adequate evaluation of the Specialized Care Center. **The committee recommends that a short-term plan (perhaps 5 years) be developed for the Specialized Care Center that would specify goals and expected outcomes.** Based on such a plan, an evaluation could then be undertaken to assess the effectiveness of the center.

COORDINATION WITH THE VA

Given that many now receiving services in the DoD health care system will eventually move to the VA health care system, it is important to have good communication between DoD and the VA. This may be particularly true in the areas of medically unexplained symptom syndromes and psychiatric disorders, where accurate diagnosis and assessment of response to treatment are important for positive patient outcomes. **The committee recommends that DoD explore ways to increase communication with the VA, particularly as it relates to the ongoing treatment of patients.**

Both patients and providers would benefit from increased educational activity regarding Persian Gulf health issues. Provider turnover within DoD is a factor that must be taken into consideration when examining the special health needs and concerns of active-duty personnel who were deployed to the Persian Gulf. Although efforts at provider education were extensive at the time the CCEP was implemented, three years have passed and many new providers have entered the system. These individuals should be oriented to the special needs, concerns, and procedures involved, and all providers should be updated regularly.

The VA has developed a number of approaches to provider education. Interactive satellite teleconferences are available periodically for medical center staff to discuss particular issues of concern. The VA conducts quarterly national telephone conference calls, directs periodic educational mailings to Persian Gulf Registry providers in each health facility, and conducts an annual conference on the health consequences of Persian Gulf service. **The committee recommends that DoD examine the activities and materials for provider education developed by the VA to determine if some of the items might be used as educational approaches for DoD providers.**

Although the topics of ongoing educational efforts are best determined by DoD on a periodic basis, **the committee recommends that DoD mount an effort designed to educate providers to the fact that conditions related to stress are not necessarily psychiatric conditions. The committee recommends that depression be a topic of education for all primary care providers, with emphasis on the facts that depression is common, it is treatable, and individuals who experience depression can continue to function.**

The committee wishes to reemphasize the fact that the CCEP is not a research protocol but rather a program designed to diagnose the health problems of those who served in the Persian Gulf. As such, information obtained through the CCEP should not be used to answer research questions. It is appropriate, however, to use the data and narrative information obtained from the CCEP to inform the clinical treatment process. In doing so, the committee believes that it is important to unbundle diagnostic categories. For example, tension headache is classified as a somatoform disorder within the category of psychiatric diagnosis.

In addition, a tremendous amount of qualitative information could be used in developing case studies to help providers better understand diagnostic and treatment approaches that appear effective at improving individual patients' conditions.

The committee recommends that CCEP information be used to develop case studies that will help educate providers about Persian Gulf health problems. There are a number of ways in which these case studies could be shared including presentation during professional meetings.

There is also a need for education and communication with individuals who were deployed to the Gulf and with their families. These individuals are concerned about the potential impact of Persian Gulf deployment on their health, whether or not their health concerns will affect their military careers, their ability to obtain health insurance once they leave the service, and a number of other issues that need to be addressed.

A variety of mechanisms are available for providing such information including individual post newsletters, the Internet, mailings to those in the Registry, and public forums. It is especially important to provide a forum for discussion each time new information is released on possible exposures. **The committee recommends that DoD develop approaches to communication and education that address the concerns of individuals deployed to the Persian Gulf and their families.**

References and Selected Bibliography

Aneshensel, CS. 1992. Social Stress: Theory and Research. *Annu Rev Socio* 18:15–38.

Aneshensel, CS. 1996. Consequences of Psychosocial Stress: The Universe of Stress Outcomes. In *Psychosocial Stress*. Academic Press, Inc.

Aneshensel, CS, Rutter, CM, and Lachenbruch, PA. 1991. Social Structure, Stress, and Mental Health: Competing Conceptual and Analytic Models. *Am Sociological Review* 56:166–178.

Barskey, AJ, Goodson, JD, Lane, RS, et al. 1988. The Amplification of Somatic Symptoms. *Psychosomatic Medicine* 50:510–519.

Bleich, A, Dycian, A, Koslowsky, M, et al. 1992. Psychiatric Implications of Missile Attacks on a Civilian Population: Israeli Lessons from the Persian Gulf War. *JAMA* 268:613–615.

Bou-Holaigah, I, Rowe, PC, and Kan, J. 1995. The Relationship Between Neurally Mediated Hypotension and the Chronic Fatigue Syndrome. *JAMA* 274:961–967.

Bremner, JD, Southwick, SM, Darnell, A, et al. 1996. Chronic PTSD in Vietnam Combat Veterans: Course of Illness and Substance Abuse. *Am J Psychiatry* 153(3):369–375.

Brody, DS, Thompson, TL, Larson, DB, et al. 1995. Recognizing and Managing Depression in Primary Care. *Gen Hosp Psych* 17:93–107.

Buchwald, D, and Garrity, D. 1994. Comparison of Patients with Chronic Fatigue Syndrome, Fibromyalgia, and Multiple Chemical Sensitivities. *Arch Intern Med* 154:2049–2053.

Calabrese, LH, Davis, ME, and Wilke, WS. 1994. Chronic Fatigue Syndrome and a Disorder Resembling Sjögren's Syndrome: Preliminary Report. *Clin Infect Dis* 18 (Suppl 1):S28–S31.

Chrousos, GP and Gold, PW. 1992. The concepts of stress and stress system disorders: Overview of physical and behavioral homeostasis. *JAMA* 267:1244–1252.

Clauw, DJ. 1995. The Pathogenesis of Chronic Pain and Fatigue Syndromes, with Special Reference to Fibromyalgia. *Med Hypotheses* 44:369–378.

Cohen, S, Tyrrell, DA, and Smith, AP. 1991. Psychological Stress and Susceptibility to the Common Cold. *N Engl J Med* 325:606–612.

Cottler, LB, Compton, WM, Mager, D, et al. 1992. Posttraumatic Stress Disorder Among Substance Users from the General Population. *Am J Psychiatry* 149:664–670.

Crum, RM, Cooper-Patrick, L, and Ford, DE. 1994. Depressive Symptoms Among General Medical Patients: Prevalence and One-Year Outcome. *Psychosom Med* 56:109–117.

Cullen, MR. 1997. Multiple Chemical Sensitivities. *Encyclopaedia of Occupational Health and Safety.*

David, A, Ferry, S, Wessely, S. 1997. Editorial. Gulf War Illness: New American Research Provides Leads but No Firm Conclusions. *BMJ* 314:239–240.

Dhabhar, FS and McEwen, BS. 1996a. Moderate Stress Enhances, and Chronic Stress Suppresses, Cell-Mediated Immunity *In Vivo*. Annual Meeting of the Soc. Neurosci 22, Abstract 536.3.

Dhabhar, FS and McEwen, BS. 1996b. Stress-Induced Enhancement of Antigen-Specific Cell-Mediated Immunity. *J Immunol* 156:2608–2615.

Dhabhar, FS, Miller, AH, McEwen, BS, and Spencer, RL. 1995. Effects of Stress on Immune Cell Distribution: Dynamics and Hormonal Mechanisms. *J Immunol* 154:5511–5527.

Eisenberg, L. 1992. Treating Depression and Anxiety in Primary Care: Closing the Gap Between Knowledge and Practice. *N Engl J Med* 326:1080–1084.

Elder, GH, Shanahan, MJ, and Clipp, EC. 1997. Linking Combat and Physical Health: The Legacy of World War II in Men's Lives. *Am J Psychiatry* 154:330–336.

Ferraccioli, G, Ghirelli, L, Scita, F, et al. 1987 EMG-Biofeedback Training in Fibromyalgia Syndrome. *J Rheumatol.* 14:820–825.

Freidman, MJ and Schnurr, PP. 1995. The Relationship Between Trauma, Post-Traumatic Stress Disorder, and Physical Health. *Neurobiological and Clinical Consequences of Stress: From Normal Adaptation to PTSD* edited by Friedman, MJ, Charney, DS, and Dutch, AY. Philadelphia: Lippincott-Raven, pp. 507–524.

Friedman, MJ, Charney, DS, and Deutch, AY. 1995. Key Questions and a Research Agenda for the Future. *Neurobiological and Clinical Consequences of Stress: From Normal Adaptation to PTSD* edited by Friedman, MJ, Charney, DS, and Deutch, AY. Philadelphia: Lippincott-Raven, pp. 527–533.

Fukuda, K, and Gantz, NM. 1995. Management Strategies for Chronic Fatigue Syndrome. *Federal Practitioner* July 1995.

Fukuda, K, Straus, SE, Hickie, I, et al. 1994. The Chronic Fatigue Syndrome: A Comprehensive Approach to Its Definition and Study. International Chronic Fatigue Study Group. *Ann Intern Med.* 121:953–959.

Goldenberg, DL, Simms, RW, Geiger, A, et al. 1990. High Frequency of Fibromyalgia in Patients with Chronic Fatigue Seen in a Primary Care Practice. *Arthritis Rheum* 33:381–387.

Goldenberg, DL. 1989. Fibromyalgia and Its Relation to Chronic Fatigue Syndrome, Viral Illness and Immune Abnormalities. *J Rheumatol* 16(Suppl 19):91–93.

Göthe, CJ, Molin, C, and Nillson, CG. 1995. The Environmental Somatization Syndrome. *Psychosomatics* 36:1–11.

Green, BL, Lindy, JD, and Grace, MC. 1994. Psychological Effects of Toxic Contamination. In *Individual and Community Responses to Trauma Disaster: The Structure of Human Chaos*. Ursano, RJ, McCaughey, BJ, and Fullerton, CJ, eds. Cambridge University Press.

Haley, RW and Kurt, TL. 1997. Self-Reported Exposure to Neurotoxic Chemical Combinations in the Gulf War: A Cross-sectional Epidemiologic Study. *JAMA* 277:231–237.

Haley, RW, Hom, J, Roland, PS, et al. 1997a. Evaluation of Neurologic Function in Gulf War Veterans. *JAMA* 277:223–230.

Haley, RW, Kurt, TL, and Hom, J. 1997b. Is There a Gulf War Syndrome? Searching for Syndromes by Factor Analysis of Symptoms. *JAMA* 277(3):215–222.

Hallman, W, and Wandersman, A. 1989. *Perception of Risk and Toxic Hazards. Psychosocial Effects of Hazardous Toxic Waste Disposal on Communities* edited by DL Peck. Springfield: Charles C. Thomas, pp. 31–56.

Helzer, JE, Robins, LN, and McEvoy, L. 1987. Post-Traumatic Stress Disorder in the General Population: Findings of the Epidemiologic Catchment Area Survey. *N Engl J Med* 317:1630–1634.

Hudson, JI, Goldenberg, DL, Pope, HG, et al. 1992. Comorbidity of Fibromyalgia with Medical and Psychiatric Disorders. *Am J Med* 92:363–367.

Hyams, KC, Wignall, S, and Roswell, R. 1996. War Syndromes and Their Evaluation: From the U.S. Civil War to the Persian Gulf War. *Ann Intern Med* 125:398–405.

IOM (Institute of Medicine). 1992. *Guidelines for Clinical Practice: From Development to Use*. Washington, DC: National Academy Press.

IOM. 1994. *Committee on the DoD Persian Gulf Syndrome Comprehensive Clinical Evaluation Program: First Report*. Washington, DC: National Academy Press.

IOM. 1995a. *Committee on the DoD Persian Gulf Syndrome Comprehensive Clinical Evaluation Program: Second Report*. Washington, DC: National Academy Press.

IOM. 1995b. *Health Consequences of Service During the Persian Gulf War: Initial Findings and Recommendations for Immediate Action*. Washington, DC: National Academy Press.

IOM. 1996a. *Evaluation of the U.S. Department of Defense Persian Gulf Comprehensive Clinical Evaluation Program*. Washington, DC: National Academy Press.

IOM. 1996b. *Health Consequences of Service During the Persian Gulf War: Recommendations for Research and Information Systems*. Washington, DC: National Academy Press.

IOM. 1997. *Adequacy of the Comprehensive Clinical Evaluation Program: Nerve Agents*. Washington, DC: National Academy Press.

Jewett, DL. 1992. Research Strategies for Investigating Multiple Chemical Sensitivity. *Toxicol Ind Health* 8:175–179.

Katon, W. 1995. Editorial: Will Improving Detection of Depression in Primary Care Lead to Improved Depressive Outcomes? *Gen Hosp Psych* 17:1–2.

Katon, W. 1996. Editorial: The Impact of Major Depression on Chronic Medical Illness. *Gen Hosp Psych* 18:215–219.

Katon, W, Von Korff, M, Lin, E, et al. 1990. Distressed High Utilizers of Medical Care: DSM-III-R Diagnoses and Treatment Needs. *Gen Hosp Psychiatry* 12:355–362.

Katon, W, Von Korff, M, Lin, E, et al. 1995. Collaborative Management to Achieve Treatment Guidelines. Impact on Depression in Primary Care. *JAMA* 273:1026–1031.

Kilburn, KH. 1993. Editorial. Symptoms, Syndrome, and Semantics: Multiple Chemical Sensitivity and Chronic Fatigue Syndrome. *Arch Environ Health* 48:368–369.

Kipen, HM. Systemic Conditions: An Introduction. *Encyclopaedia of Occupational Health and Safety*. In press.

Kipen, HM, Fiedler, N, and Lehrer, P. 1997. Multiple Chemical Sensitivities: A Primer for Pulmonologists. *Clin Pulmonary Med* 4(2):76–84.

Komaroff, AL, Fagioli, LR, Geiger, AM, et al. 1996. An Examination of the Working Class Definition of Chronic Fatigue Syndrome. *Am J Med* 100:56–64.

Koshes, RJ. 1996. The Care of Those Returned: Psychiatric Illnesses of War. In *Emotional Aftermath of the Persian Gulf War*. Ursano, RJ, and Norwood, AE, eds. Washington, DC: American Psychiatric Press.

Kroenke, K, Spitzer, RL, Williams, JB, et al. 1994. Physical Symptoms in Primary Care. Predictors of psychiatric disorders and functional impairment. *Arch Fam Med* 3:774–779.

Leonard, BE and Miller, K, eds. 1995. *Stress, the Immune System, and Psychiatry*. New York: John Wiley and Sons.

Ling, W, Compton, P, Rawon, R, and Wesson, DR.. Neuropsychiatry of Alcohol and Drug Abuse. *Neuropsychiatry*

Marmar, CR, Foy, D, Kagan, B, et al. 1993. An Integrated Approach for Treating Posttraumatic Stress. *America Psychiatric Press Review of Psychiatry* Volume 12 edited by Oldham, JM, Riba, MB, and Tasman, A. Washington, DC: Am Psychiatric Press, pp. 238–272.

Meisler, AW. 1996. Trauma, PTSD, and Substance Abuse. *PTSD Res Quarterly* 7(4):1-5.

Mellman, TA, Randolph, CA, Brawman-Mintzer, O, et al. 1992. Phenomenology and Course of Psychiatric Disorders Associated With Combat-Related Posttraumatic Stress Disorder. *Am J Psychiatry* 149(11):1568–1574.

News Release. Duke University. Dangerous Chemical Combination Presents Possible Scenario for Gulf War Illnesses.

Pokorny AD, Miller BA, Kaplan HB. 1972. The brief MAST: a shortened version of the Michigan Alcoholism Screening Test. *Am J Psychiatry* 129(3):342-345.

Reiffenberger, DH and Amundson, LH. 1996. Fibromyalgia Syndrome: A Review. *Am Fam Physician* 53(5):1698–1704.

Robbins, JM, and Kirmayer, LJ. 1996. Transient and persistent hypochrondrical worry in primary care. *Psychol Med* 26:575–589.

Rundell, JR, and Ursano, RJ. 1996. Psychiatric Responses to War Trauma. In *Emotional Aftermath of the Persian Gulf War* edited by Ursano, RJ, and Norwood, AE. Washington, DC: American Psychiatric Press, pp. 43–81.

Russell, M, Martier, S.S, Sokol, R.J, Jacobson, S, et al. 1991. Screening for pregnancy risk drinking: TWEAKING the tests. *Alcoholism Clin Exp Res* 15(2):638, 1991.

Schnall, PL, Devereux, RB, Pickering, et al. 1992. Letter. The Relationship Between "Job Strain," Workplace Diastolic Blood Pressure, and Left Ventricular Mess Index: A Correction. *JAMA* 267:1209.

Schnall, PL, Schwartz, JE, Landsbergis, PA, et al. 1992. Relation between Job Strain, Alcohol, and Ambulatory Blood Pressure. *Hypertension* 19:488–494.

Schwarts, DA, Doebbeling, BN, Merchant, JA, et al. (The Iowa Persian Gulf Study Group). 1997. Self-reported Illness and Health Status Among Gulf War Veterans. *JAMA* 277:238–245.

Simms, RW. 1994. Controlled trials of therapy in fibromyalgia syndrome. *Ballière's Clin Rheum* 8(4):917–934.

Simon, GE, Katon, WJ, and Sparks, PJ. 1990. Allergic to Life: Psychological Factors in Environmental Illness. *Am J Psychiatry* 147(7):901–906.

Sokol RJ, Martier SS, Ager JW. 1989. The T-ACE questions: practical prenatal detection of risk-drinking. *Am J Obstet Gynecol* 160(4):863-868.

Solomon, Z. 1993. *Combat Stress Reaction: The Enduring Toll of War*. New York: Plenum Press.

Southwick, SM, Morgan, A, Magy, LM, et al. 1993. Trauma-Related Symptoms in Veterans of Operation Desert Storm: A Preliminary Report. *Am J Psychiatry* 150:1524–1528.

Southwick, SM, Morgan, CA, Darnell, A, et al. 1995. Trauma-Related Symptoms in Veterans of Operation Desert Storm: A 2-Year Follow-Up. *Am J Psychiatry* 152(8):1150–1155.

Sparks, PJ, Daniell, W, Black, DW, et al. 1994a. Multiple Chemical Sensitivity Syndrome: A Clinical Perspective, I. Case Definition, Theories of Pathogenesis, and Research Needs. *J Occup Med* 36(7):718–730.

Sparks, PJ, Daniell, W, Black, DW, et al. 1994b. Multiple Chemical Sensitivity Syndrome: A Clinical Perspective, II. Evaluation, Diagnostic Testing, Treatment, and Social Considerations. *J Occup Med* 36(7):731–737.

Sutker, PB, Uddo, M, Brailey, K, et al. 1994. Psychopathology in War-Zone Deployed and Nondeployed Operation Desert Storm Troops Assigned Graves Registration Duties. *J Abnorm Psych* 103(2):383–390.

Testimony of Satu M. Somani, April 24, 1997. Gulf War Syndrome: Potential Effects of Low-Level Exposure to Sarin and/or Pyridostigmine under Conditions of Physical Stress. US House of Representatives, Government and Oversight Committee, Human Resources Subcommittee.

Testimony of Thomas N. Tiedt, April 24, 1997. Gulf War Syndrome. US House of Representatives, Government and Oversight Committee, Human Resources Subcommittee.

Testimony of Jonathon B. Tucker, April 24, 1997. Low-Level Chemical Weapons Exposures During the 1991 Persian Gulf War. US House of Representatives, Government and Oversight Committee, Human Resources Subcommittee.

The Brain: The Color of Stress. *Discover* 1997:16–20.

Ursano, RJ and Norwood, AE, eds. 1996. *Emotional Aftermath of the Persian Gulf War*. Washington, DC: American Psychiatric Press.

Ward, MH, DeLisle, H, Shores, JH, et al. 1996. Chronic fatigue complaints in primary care: Incidence and Diagnostic Patterns. *J Am Osteopath Assoc* 96:34–46.

Wearden, A and Appleby, L. 1997. Cognitive performance and complaints of cognitive impairment in chronic fatigue syndrome (CFS). *Psychol Med* 27:81–90.

Wells, KB and Burnam, MA. 1991. Caring for Depression in America: Lessons Learned from Early Findings of the Medical Outcomes Study. *Psychiatr Med* 9:503–519.

Williams, RB. 1995. Somatic Consequences of Stress. *Neurobiologial and Clinical Consequences of Stress: From Normal Adaptation to PTSD* edited by Friedman, MJ, Charney, DS, and Deutch, AY. Philadelphia: Lippincott-Raven, pp. 403–412.

Wilson, JMG and Jungner, G. 1968. *Principles and Practice of Screening for Disease*. Geneva: World Health Organization.

Wolfe, F. 1994. When to Diagnose Fibromyalgia. *Rheum Dis Clin North Am* 20:485–501.

Wolfe, F, Anderson, J, Harkness, D, et al. 1997a. A prospective, longitudinal, multicenter study of service utilization and costs in fibromyalgia. In press, *Arthritis and Rheumatism.*

Wolfe, F, Anderson, J, Harkness, D, et al. 1997b. Health Status and Disease Severity in Fibromyalgia: Results of a Six Center Longitudinal Study. In press, *Arthritis and Rheumatism.*

Wolfe, F, Anderson, J, Harkeness, D, et al. 1997c. Work and disability status of persons with fibromyalgia. *J Rheumatol* 24:1171–1178.

Wolfe, F, Ross, K, Anderson, J, et al. 1995. The Prevalence and Characteristics of Fibromyalgia in the General Population. *Arthritis Rheum* 38:19–28.

Wolfe, F, Simmons, DG, Fricton, JR, et al. 1992. The fibromyalgia and myofascial pain syndromes—a preliminary study of tender points and trigger points in persons with fibromyalgia, myofascial pain syndrome and no disease. *J Rheumatol* 19:944–951.

Wolfe, J and Proctor, SP. 1996. The Persian Gulf War: New Findings on Traumatic Exposure and Stress. *PTSD Research Quarterly* 7(1).

Wysenbeek, AJ, Shapira, Y, and Leibovici, L. 1991. Primary fibromyalgia and the chronic fatigue syndrome. *Rheumatol Int* 10:227–229.

Appendix A

Presidential Advisory Committee on Gulf War Veterans' Illnesses: Final Report Recommendations*

RECOMMENDATIONS

The Committee's evaluation of the government's response to concerns about Gulf War veterans' illnesses led us to findings in outreach, medical and clinical issues, research, chemical and biological weapons, and coordination. Based on our analyses and these findings, the Committee makes the following recommendations:

Outreach

• DOD and VA should follow the model of field-based outreach demonstrated in the Vet Centers and the Persian Gulf Family Support Program when developing health education and risk communication campaigns for active duty service members, Reserve and National Guard personnel, and other veterans. General, less specific outreach methods—e.g., hotlines and public service announcements—should be viewed as important supplements, but not as replacements.

• VA should direct its Transition Assistance Program workshop benefits counselors to specifically mention DOD and VA programs related to Gulf War veterans' illnesses.

---

*This appendix has been excerpted from the Presidential Advisory Committee on Gulf War Veterans' Illnesses report, *Presidential Advisory Committee on Gulf War Veterans' Illnesses: Final Report,* Washington, D.C.: U.S. Government Printing Office, 1996.

• VA should ensure that its initiatives under the Women Veterans Health Programs specifically provide information about Gulf War-related programs.

• VA should ensure that its outreach to Latino populations specifically provides information about Gulf War-related programs. As the Committee stated in its *Interim Report*, DOD and VA should develop and utilize more refined performance measures to determine how well outreach services are reaching concerned parties. DOD and VA officials (specifically those in the American Forces Information Service and its broadcasting arm, the Armed Forces Radio and Television Service) using media products for outreach initiatives should be aware of the difficulty in enumerating the actual readership and viewership figures and be concerned about how effectively their message saturates the targeted population.

• DOD should reissue its *Internal Information Plan* on Gulf War-related illnesses. It should make a special effort to note the revision provides the toll-free number and that individuals are encouraged to register for its Comprehensive Clinical Evaluation Program. It also should take this opportunity to provide updated information.

• In an attempt to increase veterans' and the public's awareness and understanding of the full range of the government's commitment to addressing the nature of Gulf War veterans' illnesses, DOD and VA should reevaluate the goals and objectives of their risk communication efforts. DOD and VA should develop effective methods that provide the affected community with comprehensive information concerning possible exposures to environmental hazards, potential health effects from risk factors, and explanations of ongoing and completed clinical and epidemiologic studies.

• DOD and VA should immediately develop and implement a comprehensive risk communication plan. This effort should move forward in close cooperation with agencies that have a high degree of public trust and experience with risk communication, such as the Agency for Toxic Substances and Disease Registry and the National Institute for Occupational Safety and Health.

• Because health risk information and education applies to service members who remain on active duty, members of the Reserves and National Guard, and veterans no longer in military service, DOD and VA should closely coordinate the federal government's risk communication effort for Gulf War veterans and other members of the affected community. Departmental commitments to any plan should be viewed as continuous and long-term; a sustained effort is particularly critical in light of veterans' and public skepticism arising from the recent revelations related to chemical weapons.

• In its coordinated risk communication plan, DOD and VA should engage veterans service organizations as intermediaries—and include personnel in leadership positions, such as senior enlisted personnel (for active duty military) and state veterans' service officials—in the effort to establish an efficient information exchange process where veterans receive accurate information and the departments receive valuable feedback on clinical programs, health concerns, and communication efforts.

Medical and Clinical Issues

- Given that the Food and Drug Administration's (FDA) Interim Final Rule permitting a waiver of informed consent for use of unapproved products in a military exigency is still in effect, DOD should develop enhanced orientation and training procedures to alert service personnel they may be required to take drugs or vaccines not fully approved by FDA if a conflict presents a serious threat of chemical and biological warfare.
- FDA should solicit timely public and expert comment on any rule that permits waiver of informed consent for use of investigational products in military exigencies. Among the areas that specifically should be revisited are: adequacy of disclosure to service personnel; adequacy of recordkeeping; long-term followup of individuals who receive investigational products; review by an institutional review board outside of DOD; and additional procedures to enhance understanding, oversight, and accountability.
- DOD officials at the highest echelons, including the Joint Chiefs of Staff and the Commander in Chief, should assign a high priority to dealing with the problem of lost or missing medical records. A computerized central database is important. Specialized databases must be compatible with the central database. Attention should be directed toward developing a mechanism for computerizing medical data (including classified information, if and when it is needed) in the field. DOD and VA should adopt standardized recordkeeping to ensure continuity.
- The Persian Gulf Veterans Coordinating Board and other appropriate departments and agencies should be charged to develop a protocol to implement the following recommendation, which was made in the Committee's *Interim Report*: Prior to any deployment, DOD should undertake a thorough health evaluation of a large sample of troops to enable better postdeployment medical epidemiology. Medical surveillance should be standardized for a core set of tests across all services, including timely postdeployment followup.
- VA and DOD should, in their educational outreach programs, specifically target staff members not directly involved in the care of Gulf War veterans.
- DOD and VA should include timely updates on the Comprehensive Clinical Evaluation Program or Persian Gulf Health Registry, respectively, in their Continuing Medical Education programs.

• VA and DOD should regularly brief their staffs on the Gulf War research portfolio and on the results of research studies as they become available.

• VA and DOD should regularly review staffing needs, particularly in mental health, and increase recruitment and retention of adequate numbers of medical professionals to satisfy patient needs. Staffing reviews should consider that, despite increased medical surveillance and better preventive measures, future deployments also will generate a significant number of veterans who will need care for illnesses that are difficult to diagnose.

• Since 1986, U.S. service members with certain chronic illnesses, e.g., asthma and diabetes, have been allowed to remain on active duty when regular medical monitoring is necessary. Veterans of the Gulf War with chronic illnesses are no different. Troop commanders should be reminded that adequate time off for follow-up medical appointments is a necessity and a priority.

• The government should conduct a thorough review of its policies concerning reproductive health and seek statutory authority to treat veterans and their families for service-connected problems. When indicated, genetic counseling should be provided—either via VA treatment facilities or referral—to assist veterans and their families who have reproductive concerns stemming from military service.

• The government should continue and intensify its efforts to develop stress reduction programs for all troops, with special emphasis on deployed troops.

• Since leadership and unit cohesion are so important in managing stress, DOD should specifically involve senior commanders and senior noncommissioned officers in stress management programs.

Research

• The Research Working Group of the Persian Gulf Veterans Coordinating Board should require that any proposals for new, large-scale Gulf War veterans' epidemiologic health research describe a plan to incorporate a public advisory committee into the study design, dissemination of results, or both. The Research Working Group should consider justifying a waiver of such a committee only under rare circumstances.

• The government should develop more accurate and reliable methods of recording troop locations to facilitate post-conflict health research in the future. DOD should make full use of global positioning technologies.

• The government should plan for further research on possible long-term health effects of low-level exposure to organophosphorus nerve agents such as sarin, soman, or various pesticides, based on studies of groups with well-characterized exposures, including: (a) cases of U.S. workers exposed to organophosphorus pesticides; and (b) civilians exposed to the chemical warfare agent sarin during the 1994 and 1995 terrorist attacks in Japan. Additional work should include followup and evaluation of an appropriate subset of any U.S. service personnel who are presumed to be exposed during the Gulf War. The government should begin by consulting with appropriate experts, both governmental and nongovernmental, on organophosphorus nerve agent effects. Studies of human populations with well-characterized exposures will be much more revealing than studies based on animal models, which should be given lower priority.

- Since a number of Gulf War risk factors are potential human carcinogens that could result in increased rates of cancer beginning decades after exposure, VA should continue to monitor Gulf War veterans through its ongoing mortality study for increased rates of lung, liver, and other cancers.
- Depleted uranium munitions are likely to be used in future conflicts involving U.S. service personnel. To fully elucidate the health effects of depleted uranium munitions, VA should conduct research that compares the health status of individuals with embedded fragments of DU shrapnel with appropriate control groups.
- The government should continue to collect and archive serum samples from U.S. service personnel when feasible.
- The Research Working Group should more thoroughly consult with other federal agencies with relevant expertise—such as the National Institutes of Health (particularly the National Institute of Environmental Health Sciences) and the Agency for Toxic Substances and Disease Registry—on basic, clinical, and epidemiologic research and on risk communication.

Chemical and Biological Weapons

- All U.S. service personnel assigned to units near the Khamisiyah demolition activity should be notified and encouraged to enroll in VA's Persian Gulf Health Registry or DOD's Comprehensive Clinical Evaluation Program. In determining the extent of possible chemical warfare agent exposure at Khamisiyah and any other sites that future investigations uncover, the government should use the best theoretical and practical assessment tools available. The Committee recognizes the large number of variables that can affect the outcome of any determination, but identifies the following as essential principles:

  — Where objective, unrebutted evidence suggests the release of chemical warfare agents in the vicinity of U.S. troops, every effort should be made to identify the source of the agent and to model

the downwind footprint of the potential distribution of agent at the general population exposure level (or lower threshold, if appropriate);
— When a downwind footprint is established, a conservative, presumptive-exposure area should be defined that reflects the uncertainties of the modeling effort. The presumptive-exposure area should, at a minimum, include all sites within a circle that has a radius equal to the length of the downwind footprint; and
— Troops within the presumptive-exposure area should be notified and encouraged to enroll in the CCEP or Registry.

- All reports of positive M256 kits and Fox detections must be thoroughly investigated. Where unit logs record positive detections by either type of equipment, members of that unit should be notified and encouraged to enroll in VA's Persian Gulf Health Registry or DOD's Comprehensive Clinical Evaluation Program.
- To ensure credibility and thoroughness, further investigation of possible chemical or biological warfare agent exposures during the Gulf War should be conducted by a group independent of DOD. Openness in oversight activities—including public access to information and veteran participation—public notice of meetings, opportunity for public comment, and regular reporting are essential. Full public accountability is critical.

Coordination

- A Presidential Review Directive (PRD) should be issued to instruct the National Science and Technology Council to develop an interagency plan to address health preparedness for and readjustment of veterans and families after future conflicts and peacekeeping missions. The President's Committee of Advisors on Science and Technology and other nongovernmental experts, as appropriate, should be asked to review the plan 12 months after the PRD is issued and again at 18 months to ensure national expertise is brought to bear on these issues.

Appendix B

Health Consequences of Service During the Persian Gulf War: Initial Findings and Recommendations for Immediate Action*

FINDINGS AND RECOMMENDATIONS

In this report, the IOM Committee has attempted to highlight issues we believe would benefit from immediate action. In reviewing the large volume of documents and the progress of research currently underway, we have identified areas that need prompt attention. As the scope and extent of health problems of Persian Gulf veterans have appeared to expand, the social response also has grown. The committee believes that this has resulted in a fragmented attempt to solve these problems. Thus we believe that sustained, coordinated, and serious efforts must be made in the near term to focus both the medical, social, and research response of the Government and of individuals and researchers. Hence, the findings and recommendations that follow are offered with the intent to focus and sharpen the debate, and to improve the quality of the data, and thereby, scientific inference. Finally, we hope to impact in a positive way the health in persons who served in the Persian Gulf War, as well as in those who may follow in other military encounters.

Recommendations for immediate action follow based on the findings presented here and the background information presented in the next chapter. The recommendations are to be viewed as independent, and are not presented in any priority order within categories. The recommendations are divided into

---

*This appendix was excerpted from the Institute of Medicine report *Health Consequences of Service During the Persian Gulf War: Initial Findings and Recommendations for Immediate Action,* Washington, D.C.: National Academy Press, 1995.

three categories: data and databases, coordination/process, and considerations of study design needs.

DATA AND DATABASES

Finding I

The VA Persian Gulf Health Registry is not a population database and is not administered uniformly, therefore, it cannot serve the purposes of research into the etiology or treatment of possible health problems. The Committee recognizes that certain tabulated descriptions of affected persons may legitimately be carried out for reasons other than the generation of scientific data. Specifically, there may be medical reasons for collecting information about patients with certain kinds of problems, especially diagnostic problems, particularly in medical settings where the information may be subjected to more intense scrutiny. An example is the establishment of the VA referral centers for Gulf War veterans. Since a limited number of veterans have been referred to these centers, and because the sample is self-selected, the Committee concludes that it is unlikely that productive scientific research (especially of an epidemiological nature) can ever be based on the data generated by the referral centers or the health registry as currently organized.

Recommendations

- The VA Persian Gulf Health Registry should be limited and specific to gathering information to determine the types of conditions reported. The role of this registry should be clearly defined as a means for identifying and reporting illnesses among Gulf War veterans with concerns about their health. There should be efforts to implement quality control and standardization of data collected by the registry from other VA facilities. The VA registry data should not be promoted or described as a means to determine prevalence estimates or identify the etiology of a disease, but should be reviewed promptly for enrollment trends and potential sentinel events.
- The VA should improve publicity regarding the existence of the Persian Gulf Health Registry, and encourage all concerned PGW veterans to be registered.
- Where possible the referral centers, standardized protocol should be used in each VA facility.
- The timeliness of data received from the VA Medical Centers (VAMC) to be entered into the PG Health Registry database needs to be improved.

Finding 2

No single comprehensive data system exists that enables researchers to track the health of Persian Gulf War veterans both while on active duty and after separation. As a result, it is not possible to conduct research and determine the morbidity and mortality experience of this population. Although both the VA and the DoD have medical records systems in place, they are inadequate and unlinked. This lack of a single data system is a hindrance to research concerning delayed health effects, both for Persian Gulf veterans and for those serving in future encounters.

Recommendation

- The Vice President of the United States should chair a committee composed of representatives from HHS, DoD, and VA to devise a plan to link data systems on health outcomes with the development of standardized health forms, the ability to access information rapidly, and an organized system of records for rapid entry into the data system.

Finding 3

The characteristics of the population at risk are critical to any definitive studies of Gulf War health effects. The DoD has taken the proper steps to enumerate and describe this population that will be part of the planned, but yet incomplete, Army Geographical Information System model.

Recommendations

- The DoD registry needs to be completed as quickly and accurately as possible.
- The Secretaries of DoD and VA should develop a single service-connected health record, for each present active duty and former service member. All health data entries should be recorded in this single record for the individual.

COORDINATION/PROCESS

Finding 4

The committee has noted with interest and some concern the wide variety of disciplines and expertise among persons who have considered possible causes of a mystery illness. It has appeared to the committee that some of these persons and organizations are simply not qualified to draw reasoned scientific conclusions, or to implement those conclusions by means of specific medical intervention. There may be substantial risk from inappropriate interventions because of adverse reactions to drugs, development of resistant strains of microorganisms, or especially the diversion of attention away from more orthodox diagnoses and treatments that hold some promise of relief from symptoms of a "mystery illness."

Recommendation

- Decisions to provide funding, to refer patients, or to change usual operating procedures for providing financial support should be based on more solid scientific bases than has sometimes been evident in prior resource allocation. Funding should be subject to external peer review and approval.

Finding 5

There are dozens of studies of PGW health effects underway now, and many others are being initiated. Several efforts appear to be redundant, yet there are clearly gaps where research efforts are necessary. In its final report, the IOM Committee will recommend some additional specific research projects.

Presently, the total number of undiagnosed conditions is unknown because the data either are insufficiently understood or unavailable. Data that are available are fragmented, managed by different methods in different agencies, and based on a wide variety of unconnected rationales, from both military and civilian institutions. Many research efforts should, but do not, rely on a common set of data resources. Because so many unanswered questions remain concerning multi-system etiologies that have been proposed to explain undiagnosed signs and symptoms, all future as well as current evaluations must ensure that findings can be reconciled across studies.

Recommendations

- The Persian Gulf Veterans Coordinating Board (chaired by the Secretaries of VA, DoD, HHS) should actively coordinate all studies developed from any new initiatives that receive federal funding, to prevent unnecessary duplication and to assure that high priority recommended studies be conducted. These studies should undergo appropriate external peer review before, during, and after data collection and analysis.
- More staff should be assigned by the Persian Gulf Veterans Coordinating Board in order to monitor, collect, assemble, and make accessible when appropriate all relevant requested emerging data from studies now underway, and make periodic reports to the appropriate federal oversight authority.
- Each new initiative should be evaluated in the context of what it can contribute. That is, each new study should add something of value to the information already being obtained or accumulated.

CONSIDERATIONS OF STUDY DESIGN NEEDS

Finding 6

To date, most studies of PGW veterans have been piecemeal—one military unit here, one collection of volunteers with some problem there, etc. But, some of these studies have several fundamental problems. They are necessarily incomplete, they usually lack proper controls, they are hard to generalize, they are subject to grave statistical problems because of post-hoc hypotheses and multiple comparisons, and where an effect truly exists they tend to have low statistical power to detect a difference. Thus, bits and pieces are not likely to answer any critical questions. The committee recognizes that an initial effort to survey a sample of veterans is underway, but more is needed.

Overall, there has been a broad and serious lack of adequate attention to the design of individual studies, and even more seriously, the scope and organization of an appropriate collection of studies, each focused on the resolution of a specific question. The committee regards this as a grave, though understandable failure. Experts in research design can and should work shoulder to shoulder with experts in the subject matter of each individual study; this is particularly true for work in epidemiology. A broader view of the whole collection of studies, including input from experts in subject matter and in research methods, persons knowledgeable about data sources and medical care systems, and those with general appreciation of public concerns and public policy, has been conspicuously lacking. We believe that good studies could be done, but that they will require substantial input from experts in epidemiological methods.

Recommendations

• The VA and DoD should determine the *specific* research questions that need to be answered. Epidemiologic studies should be designed with the objective of answering these questions given the input of experts in epidemiologic research methods and data analysis, along with the input of experts in the subject matter areas to be investigated.

• To obtain data on symptom prevalence, health status, and diagnosed disease, the Secretaries of DoD and VA should collaborate to conduct a population-based survey of persons who served in the PG, and of PG-era service personnel. The study should be designed to allow for adequate comparisons of outcome by sex, service branch, and rank, with oversampling among certain subgroups to allow for analysis. The IOM committee is willing to comment on and assist in the study design. An evaluation of the feasibility and need for a longitudinal study should take place coincident with this national survey.

Finding 7

Initial characterizations of smoke and unburned contaminants from the oil well fires and other sources are not adequate, nor have the data available been reduced to a format usable for drawing conclusions or conducting health studies. Considerable data exist from a wide number of sources, but they have not been compiled or analyzed in any organized or efficient way. For example, lead levels that would cause acute toxicity have been reported; however, questions about the validity of these reports have not been adequately addressed.

Recommendations

• DoD should assemble and organize these data from all sources for evaluation by the IOM committee.

• DoD should conduct a study that simulates exposure in tents heated by diesel fuel, with composition similar to that used in the PG. Fuels and conditions should simulate as closely as possible the conditions that existed in the PG. Exposure to lead and its possible effects should be explored further. The committee reviewed work done indicating that some personnel in the Gulf had lead levels consistent with acute intoxication. Thus in investigating lead exposure, special attention should be given to any history of abdominal pain or mental disorders.

Finding 8

As acknowledged by the investigator, the VA study of mortality in the PG veteran population is of insufficient duration to observe a higher rate of death than would be expected from chronic disease outcomes.

Recommendation

- The VA should plan and provide support for its mortality study to continue in the future in order to permit the detection and investigation of long-term mortality from chronic disease.

Finding 9

Although infertility, unrecognized and recognized pregnancy loss, premature delivery, fetal growth retardation, birth defects, and abnormal development are all components of reproductive health, studies and surveillance efforts to date have focused primarily on birth defects, fetal and neonatal deaths, and low birth weight. Adverse reproductive effects can be mediated through males as well as females, so it is important to study exposures of both parents. Information on infertility and miscarriage has not been included in the VA Health Registry efforts. Moreover, data on outcomes are available only from a single cluster study in Mississippi and the Army Surgeon General's preliminary data evaluation. DoD launched recently a study of reproductive health, and the VA and DoD clinical evaluation protocols provide some surveillance of infertility, miscarriage, birth defects, and infant deaths.

The design of scientific studies to address reproductive risk associated with environmental exposures is complex. A variety of endpoints may occur throughout the continuum beginning with fertility, through intrauterine, peripartum, and neonatal development, and continuing with effects manifested only later in childhood. Additionally, sophisticated expertise is required to document environmental exposures as the etiology for adverse pregnancy experience. There are research groups in some academic and federal settings that could, if deemed appropriate, conduct such complex research.

Recommendations

- VA and DoD should include reproductive outcomes among the array of health endpoints in surveillance programs based on medical records and individual questionnaires. Medical records, such as those to be included in the Seabees reproductive study and the DoD reproductive health study, would be suitable to ascertain stillbirth, low birth weight, preterm delivery, and major birth defects. Questionnaires such as those administered for the VA health registry exam could, in addition, address questions of infertility and clinically recognized miscarriage.

- The Persian Gulf Veterans Coordinating Board should consider specific exposures that are most likely to adversely affect reproductive health of women, men or both, distinguishing between agents that would affect reproductive health only if exposure occurred at or around the time of critical periods during pregnancy versus those that might have effects that would persist after the cessation of exposure. As specific hypotheses linking exposure and reproductive outcomes are identified, studies that are suitable to providing more conclusive results for those associations should be designed.
- The Persian Gulf Veterans Coordinating Board should remain alert but skeptical about cluster studies such as those underway in Mississippi. Studies of this kind may be valuable in suggesting etiologic hypotheses; however, they have little promise for resolving questions about links between experiences in the Persian Gulf and reproductive health. Population-based studies of reproductive health outcomes are essential to resolve questions of effects of Persian Gulf War service.

Finding 10

Women who did not realize that they were pregnant at the time were deployed to the Gulf; others became pregnant during their service in the Gulf. These groups of women may have been exposed to substances potentially hazardous to themselves and to their unborn babies. A study would permit comparisons of birth outcomes and potential adverse health effects on women exposed at different times in their pregnancies.

Recommendation

- The Persian Gulf Veterans Coordinating Board should conduct a study to compare women deployed to the PG who were or who became pregnant at any time during the Persian Gulf War with an appropriate group of other women who were pregnant, but did not serve in the PGW, to evaluate potential adverse health outcomes to the mother or child. This study should only be done if a sufficient number of women can be identified. Efforts should be made to gather exposure information relevant to service at potentially high-risk times during gestation.

Finding 11

The committee has become aware that rosters exist that contain the names of persons vaccinated with anthrax and botulinum toxoid.

Recommendation

- DoD should maintain its lists of those receiving anthrax and botulinum vaccines for the purpose of conducting follow-up studies on these cohorts.

Finding 12

Troops were given packets of pyridostigmine bromide (PB) pills to be taken as a prophylactic to the threat of nerve agent exposure, at the direction of their commanding officer. PB by itself, in recommended doses, is a safe drug. Additionally, DEET (*N,N*-diethyl-*m*-toluamide) and permethrin were used by the troops to prevent insect bites. There is some information about the possible long-term toxicity to humans of DEET absorbed through the skin; however there appears to be little or no information about dermal absorption of permethrin from residues left on clothing, bedding, or elsewhere. Although permethrin is generally not applied to skin, animal studies have shown that permethrin is transferred from cloth to skin, and subsequently absorbed (NRC, 1994). There is little information about how PB, DEET, and permethrin might interact; interactions among these compounds are possible and are inadequately studied.

Recommendation

- Studies are needed to resolve uncertainties about whether PB, DEET, and permethrin have additive or synergistic effects. Unsubstantiated suggestions that they may have chronic neurotoxic effects need to be tested in carefully controlled studies in appropriate animal models. Appropriate laboratory animal studies of interactions between DEET, PB, and permethrin should be conducted.

Finding 13

Reported symptoms suggestive of visceral leishmanial infections include fever, chronic fatigue, malaise, cough, intermittent diarrhea, abdominal pain, weight loss, anemia, lymphadenopathy, and splenomegaly. The committee has considered two aspects of exposure to *L. tropica* and resulting infection with leishmania: the occurrence of either cutaneous or visceral leishmaniasis; and the possibility that some component of the poorly defined illness referred to as "Gulf War Syndrome" may result from leishmania infection.

Leishmaniasis (*L. tropica*) in PGW veterans has been evaluated in some very limited clinical studies, but not in epidemiological studies. The clinical studies suggest that the complex of symptoms in the PGW veterans diagnosed with leishmaniasis differs from what has been described in the literature for other forms of leishmaniasis. A major limitation to further investigation and diagnosis of leishmaniasis is the lack of an informative serologic test or other easy to use screening tests.

Recommendations

- The DoD Joint Technology Coordination Group II has research responsibilities for infectious diseases of military importance and should give high priority to the development of a screening approach to be used under field conditions expected in deployment, and a useful diagnostic test for *L. tropica.* The board also should review the status of leishmania research, with a view toward either drafting a request for proposals for test development, or the structured coordination of existing activities.
- All physicians should be notified to look for symptoms that are consistent with both leishmania infection and those reported as "Gulf War Syndrome" Clear instructions for follow-up actions should be widely communicated through the physician community. Veterans of Desert Storm should be notified that if they have symptoms that may suggest viscerotropic leishmaniasis they should bring this possibility to the attention of the staff at any facility where they obtain any health care, whether it is in the VA system or not. The latter may be particularly important due to the potential for long-term survival of leishmania in the host.
- When it becomes feasible, VA, DoD, or both should conduct an epidemiologic and seroepidemiologic study of leishmaniasis in PGW veterans presenting symptoms or conditions and appropriate controls. Special attention should center on a possible relation between leishmaniasis and the "Gulf War Syndrome."

Finding 14

The ecology and epidemiology of *L. tropica* are insufficiently studied. Many important questions remain unanswered concerning host species, vectors, and means of transmission to military personnel. The possible role of dogs as reservoirs of disease and the existence of vectors other than sand flies are questions that have been raised.

Recommendations

- DoD should closely monitor all information regarding ecological and clinical studies of *L. tropica* being conducted in the U.S. and abroad.
- International and U.S. researchers should be queried concerning any advances in diagnostic techniques for identifying *L. tropica.*

Appendix C

Health Consequences of Service During the Persian Gulf War: Recommendations for Research and Information Systems*

CHARGE TO THE COMMITTEE: ITS FINDINGS AND RECOMMENDATIONS

Overview

In this chapter we summarize the findings and principal recommendations of the Committee to Review the Health Consequences of Service During the Persian Gulf War (PGW). Most of the findings are discussed at greater length in the chapters that follow.

Our task was to respond to three specific charges. Each finding is linked to at least one of the charges, and for each we note the principal connection. Recommendations follow each of the findings. The committee was charged as follows:

---

*These findings and recommendations were taken from the Institute of Medicine report, *Health Consequences of Service During the Persian Gulf War: Recommendations for Research and Information Systems,* Washington, D.C.: National Academy Press, 1996.

THE COMMITTEE'S CHARGE

Charge 1

> Assess the effectiveness of actions taken by the Secretary of Veterans Affairs and the Secretary of Defense to collect and maintain information that is potentially useful for assessing the health consequences of military service referred to subsection (a) [of PL 102-585, Persian Gulf (PG) theater of operations during the PGW].

The committee makes four recommendations (recommendations 13–16) in this report regarding the collection and maintenance of information that is potentially useful for assessing the health consequences of military service in the PGW. These recommendations support completion of certain data sets, prompt reporting of research findings and submission for publication in peer-reviewed journals, strengthened medical and epidemiologic research capabilities of the armed forces, and strengthening the decision-making processes for study selection.

Charge 2

> Make recommendations on means of improving the collection and maintenance of such information.

The committee makes five recommendations (recommendations 1, 4, and 8–10) on the collection and maintenance of information on the health consequences of service in the PG. We also give considerable attention to information systems that would be useful in future conflicts. These recommendations are based largely on experience with systems in place for the PGW that have shown some gaps and defects that can be remedied.

Charge 3

> Make recommendations as to whether there is [a] sound scientific basis for an epidemiologic study or studies of the health consequences of such service, and if the recommendation is that there is [a] sound scientific basis for such a study or studies, the nature of the study or studies.

The committee believes that there is indeed a sound basis for epidemiologic studies, and eight recommendations follow (recommendations 2, 3, 5–7, and 11–13).[1] However, the committee does not recommend an additional nationwide epidemiologic study of PG veterans, because such a study is likely to be of limited scientific value at this time. Those large studies that are currently under way should be completed as quickly as possible, while meeting high scientific standards, including a high response rate and a thorough investigation of potential biases, as recommended below.

FINDINGS AND RECOMMENDATIONS

Finding

Recent military deployments, especially in Vietnam and in the Persian Gulf, have demonstrated that concerns about the health consequences of participation in military action may arise long after deployment has ended and that the evaluation of those concerns and the provision of health care to affected personnel may present formidable challenges both to epidemiologists and to medical caregivers. Although some of these challenges can be attributed to the intrinsic difficulty of evaluating poorly understood clusters of events that were not among the expected consequences of combat or of environmental conditions, they also may be attributed in part to limitations of the systems used to collect and manage data regarding the health and service-related exposures of military personnel. No system of record keeping can be expected to provide the information needed to address every unanticipated research issue, including those regarding the health consequences of military service. Nevertheless, the committee has identified several possible improvements in the systems and practices for collecting information on the health and service-related exposures of military personnel. Such changes would increase the ability of the military services to pursue appropriate investigations in the future. Such changes also would increase the capacity of the services to evaluate the efficacy of mobilization-supporting health services (including approaches and methodologies for disease prevention employed before, during, and after mobilization) and would aid in providing the best possible medical care to military service personnel and veterans (Charge 2).

Recommendation 1. The Department of Defense (DoD), the branches of the armed services, and the Department of Veterans Affairs (DVA)

---

[1] Recommendation 13 has been counted as applicable to both Charge 1 and Charge 3, and therefore appears with both.

should continue to work together to develop, fund, and staff medical information systems that include a single, uniform, continuous, and retrievable electronic medical record for each service person. The uniform record should include each relevant health item (including baseline personal risk factors, every inpatient and outpatient medical contact, and all health-related interventions), allow linkage to exposure and other data sets, and have the capability to incorporate relevant medical data from beyond DoD and DVA institutions (e.g., U.S. Public Health Service facilities, civilian medical providers, and other health care institutions). Appropriate consent and protection of individual privacy must be considered for information obtained and included.

Finding

The number and variety of studies regarding consequences of the PGW are already considerable. To date, most health-related studies specifically involving PGW veterans have focused on short-term mental health consequences of deployment, the role of combat exposure, and other stressors experienced in the theater of operations and, to a lesser extent, on problems relating to demobilization and readjustment to civilian life among reservist and National Guard personnel. A few reports have included limited longitudinal follow-up data concerning men and women who served in the PG. Important information may be gained through longer follow-up of some of these groups, particularly since at least one of these groups was first to arrive in the theater, and precombat data are available. Also needed are studies of risk factors in modern deployments predictive of combat stress reactions, posttraumatic stress disorder (PTSD), and other psychiatric disorders of military personnel and veterans. Studies relevant to the trauma of war and the ensuing mental health consequences should concentrate special attention on improving efforts in prevention, intervention, and follow-up (Charge 3).

Recommendation 2. The DoD and DVA should conduct further studies, with appropriate statistical and epidemiological support, to identify risk factors for stress-related psychiatric disorders among military personnel (active and reserve) and to develop better methods to buffer and ameliorate the psychiatric consequences of modern training, deployment, combat, demobilization, and return to daily living.

Recommendation 3. Studies being conducted by DoD and DVA that have included longitudinal follow-up of the mental health of veterans who served in the PG should be supported with continued follow-up after appropriate peer review of study methods. Follow-up in these studies should be sufficient to provide at least a decade of information comparing the mental health status of those deployed with those not deployed.

Finding

The military dominance of U.S. forces in the PGW increased the relative significance of physical and natural environmental exposures as important sources of potential morbidity and mortality, compared with combat injuries. This is likely to recur in future deployments (Charge 2).

Recommendation 4. The DoD should ensure that military medical preparedness for deployments includes detailed attempts to monitor natural and man-made environmental exposures and to prepare for rapid response, early investigation, and accurate data collection, when possible, on physical and natural environmental exposures that are known or possible in the specific theater of operations.

Finding

National Guard and reserve component personnel may differ substantially from active duty personnel in average age, level of training, occupational specialties, family status, and readiness for deployment. Further, it is unclear whether either policies and procedures or the manner in which they are implemented differs between activated reserve or National Guard units and active duty troops for mobilization, deployment, demobilization, and return. All of these factors may affect the health consequences of deployment (Charge 3).

Recommendation 5. Research is needed to determine whether differences in personal characteristics or differences in policies and procedures for mobilization, deployment, demobilization, and return of reserves, National Guard, and regular troops are associated with different or adverse health consequences. If there are associations, strategies necessary to prevent or reduce these adverse health effects should be developed.

Finding

Completed studies have described the mortality experience of troops deployed to the PG during the period of deployment and in the 2-year period after deployment. These studies have documented a consistent pattern of increased risk of death from unintentional injury for the cohort of deployed troops compared with those not deployed to the PG. However, death rates from disease were not significantly increased. Continued monitoring and further study of mortality rates among veterans of the PGW will be of value in assessing the long-term health consequences of deployment (Charge 3).

Recommendation 6. The mortality experience of PG veterans should continue to be monitored for as long as 30 years, on a regular basis, including comparisons with that of PG-era veterans. (PG-era veterans have been defined as those in military service at the time of the PGW, but assigned or deployed elsewhere.) Research investigators should focus on the reported excess mortality from unintentional injury, on mortality from specific illnesses, and on evidence of elevation (or reduction) in the risk of death from other causes.

Recommendation 7. The DVA should exert greater effort to improve understanding of the reasons for excess mortality from unintentional injury. Detailed evaluation is needed beyond death certificate data concerning the circumstances surrounding fatal injury through more focused case-control studies to identify both individual risk factors and remediable causes.

Finding

The armed services and the DVA together are developing a shared basic epidemiological data system, the Defense Medical Epidemiological Database (DMED) (Charge 2).

Recommendation 8. The DMED system should be continued, expanded as planned, expedited to develop the proposed integrated information management system, linked to other key systems, and evaluated regularly.

Finding

Considerable effort has been devoted by DoD to the development of a Troop Exposure Assessment Model (TEAM) for describing the PGW experience of veterans. This has included the completion of an information system designed to establish the geographic location of each unit from January 15, 1991, until the unit departed from the Gulf theater. This system has the potential to be linked to data on regional environmental conditions but will necessarily be devoid of most individual data (such as pesticide exposure or individual health risk factors) (Charge 2).

Recommendation 9. The DoD should complete development of information systems to expeditiously and directly pinpoint unit locations at a high level of disaggregation in space and time (that is, fine detail) and to document local environmental conditions, including appropriate data quality checks, with direct data entry into the system. There is likely to be a need for a similar information system during and after any future conflict, and DoD should prepare and continually update plans for such a nonpaper system. A manual for use of the information systems by research investigators should be compiled, with the strengths and limitations identified.

Finding

The power and complexity of analyses based on space-time geographical information system (GIS) data require careful attention to data quality and the limits imposed by various data items. Quality improvement and assessment of limits are continuous processes and depend on detailed evaluation of data needs for specific analytic questions (Charge 2).

Recommendation 10. For every specific question posed to the current TEAM, DoD should assess the strengths and limitations of the TEAM as a resource for evaluating the health significance of geographically defined exposures of troops, including those in the PGW and those in conflicts that may develop in the future. Evaluations and recommendations for possible modification of the TEAM should be reported to the PG Coordinating Board, Research Working Group.

Finding

Given the unprecedented numbers of women serving in the PG, especially those in largely new roles, including combat support, it is important to specially evaluate the health consequences and needs for health services of women who served in the PG. Preliminary findings from studies being conducted at the Boston VA Medical Center (VAMC) indicate that additional research in this area is needed. Additional research is also needed on the health effects of having male and female personnel serve together in combat or under threat of combat (Charge 3).

> **Recommendation 11.** The DoD and DVA should ensure that studies of the health effects of deployment, including effects on PGW veterans, include evaluation of exposures, experiences, and situations of both women and men, with attention to their age, prior military service, marital and parental status, and other gender-specific parameters.
>
> **Recommendation 12.** The DoD and DVA should conduct studies of the health consequences of assigning men and women to serve together in combat or under the threat of enemy action. Such work should be undertaken with a focus on prevention and amelioration of any added stresses.

Finding

Several important studies are currently under way. Worthwhile data are being collected and prepared, and the studies should be completed promptly, with the necessary personnel and funding to collect the additional data needed, to conduct appropriate analyses, and to evaluate potential biases. Findings from these studies are likely to provide leads as to whether or not additional research along these lines is required to produce more specific findings (Charges 1 and 3).

- The Naval Health Research Center at San Diego has undertaken a series of studies under the general title of "Epidemiologic Studies of Morbidity Among Gulf War Veterans: A Search for Etiologic Agents and Risk Factors." These studies hold promise for answering some important questions about the health of PGW veterans after demobilization and about the possibility that veterans and their spouses may experience an excess risk of adverse pregnancy outcomes as a result of service in the PGW. The studies are being carried out with care, excellent planning, and proper pilot efforts to determine feasibility.

Upon completion, these studies should provide important guidance concerning whether veterans have experienced hospitalization at rates in excess of their nondeployed peers, have developed specific symptoms or illnesses related to their PGW experience, or have experienced risks that have resulted in adverse reproductive outcomes related to their service in the Gulf.

Recommendation 13a. The Naval Health Research studies in San Diego should be completed and results published as designed and scheduled.

• Although there are significant problems with the DVA National Health Survey, the investigators have designed additional phases of the study that will be important to complete. The physical examinations and follow-up of nonrespondents to the mail survey will be an important step toward describing potential biases and evaluating signs and symptoms of both PG and PG-era study participants.

Recommendation 13b. The DVA National Health Survey should be completed and results published as designed and scheduled.

• The DVA-DoD study that was designed to examine predictors of enrollment in the DVA PG Health Registry (PGHR) may provide useful information as to what objectively measurable factors contribute to self-selection into the registry. In addition to the proposed analysis of associations among demographics, past health experiences, and health behaviors as possible predictors of enrollment, information on the eligibility of individuals for health care, as well as the type of health care, could generate additional hypotheses to be investigated.

Recommendation 13c. Evaluation of predictors of enrollment in the DVA PGHR should be promptly completed and results published. Included, if possible, should be information on type of care requested, required, and received.

Finding

The armed forces have had small but high-quality and effective capabilities in epidemiology. Recent cutbacks have reduced these capabilities, with potentially serious effects on both military preparedness and the health care of veterans. The Theater Area Medical Laboratory (TAML) is an example of how specialists can respond rapidly to potential health problems of troops deployed in various areas of the world and provide immediate and useful information necessary to maintain the military readiness of the armed forces. In addition, well-trained epidemiologists and preventive medicine specialists are necessary for conducting the relevant population-based epidemiologic studies, with comprehensive exposure assessment, that have the greatest likelihood of being informative about the health consequences of any future deployment. Such capability should permit studies that extend beyond the time of an individual's active duty service and that are capable of responding to questions of delayed effects that may emerge only years, or even decades, after a military operation (Charge 1).

> **Recommendation 14.** The epidemiologic capabilities of the armed forces should be strengthened rather than reduced. The command structure should be kept informed about the reasons for and the results of this recommendation and its relevance to military preparedness and effectiveness, and should be encouraged to support appropriate epidemiologic work in the theater of operations and in the postdeployment period.

Finding

Much good work on symptom complexes and other matters discussed in this report has been done by DoD, DVA, and their contractors. However, it is evident from the references cited in this report that many are in the "gray literature"—available to those who know they exist and how to ask for them, but not published in the open, peer-reviewed scientific literature where they will be fully indexed and readily available, with some assurance that they meet at least minimal scientific standards. Even this committee, with the contacts and expertise it developed over time, had difficulty in identifying and obtaining some of these reports. The committee also is concerned about the high cost of much recent research and the necessity for maximizing the nation's overall return on that investment. In summary, the committee believes that health-related research is not finalized until it is published and readily accessible in peer-reviewed journals (Charge 1).

> **Recommendation 15.** The DoD and DVA should adopt a policy that internal and contract-supported reports on health research will be submitted for publication in the peer-reviewed scientific literature in a timely manner.

Finding

Some research directed toward reports of unexplained illnesses after the PGW was flawed in the questions posed, populations studied, or research design. We believe that these defects could have been identified before research projects were funded if requests for proposals had been announced generally and had been open to the scientific community at large and if fully developed research proposals had been reviewed by panels of qualified expert peers. Some research was announced and reviewed in this manner, but much more could be so treated, to the benefit of both veterans and the public (Charge 1).

Recommendation 16. The Congress, DVA, and DoD should adopt a policy that unless there are well-specified, openly stated reasons to the contrary, requests for proposals for research related to unexplained illnesses or other needed health-related research will be publicly announced and open to the scientific community at large, that proposals will be reviewed by panels of appropriately qualified experts, and that funding will follow the recommendations of those experts.

Appendix D

Evaluation of the U.S. Department of Defense Persian Gulf Comprehensive Clinical Evaluation Program: Overall Assessment and Recommendations*

1.) OVERALL ASSESSMENT OF THE CCEP GOALS PROCEDURES:

The Comprehensive Clinical Evaluation Program (CCEP) clinical protocol is a thorough, systematic approach to the diagnosis of a wide spectrum of diseases. A specific medical diagnosis or diagnoses can be reached for most patients by using the CCEP protocol. The Department of Defense (DoD) has made conscientious efforts to build consistency and quality assurance into this program at the many medical treatment facilities (MTFs) and regional medical centers (RMCs) across the country.

The committee is impressed with the quality of the design and the efficiency of the implementation of the clinical protocol, the considerable devotion of resources to this program, and the remarkable amount of work that has been accomplished in a year. The high professional standards, commitment, and diligence of the physicians involved in the CCEP at the RMCs were readily apparent at the three committee meetings. The committee commends the DoD for its efforts to provide high-quality medical care in the CCEP and the success that it has achieved to date in developing the infrastructure necessary to efficiently contact, schedule, refer, and track thousands of patients through the system.

Overall, the systematic, comprehensive set of clinical practice guidelines set forth in the CCEP are appropriate, and they have assisted physicians in the determination of specific diagnoses for thousands of patients across the country.

---

*This appendix is excerpted from the Institute of Medicine report, *Evaluation of the U.S. Department of Defense Persian Gulf Comprehensive Clinical Evaluation,* Washington, D.C.: National Academy Press, 1996.

2.) GENERAL RECOMMENDATIONS FOR THE IMPLEMENTATION OF THE CCEP:

2.1.) Referrals of Patients from Phase I to Phase II of the CCEP:

2.1.1.) Structure and revise the CCEP protocol and logistics to allow the majority of patients to receive a final diagnosis by Phase I:

Currently, the majority of patients do not receive a final diagnosis until Phase II, yet some of these patients have straightforward medical problems. The Committee recommends that final diagnoses could be reached in Phase I if more diagnostic resources are made available. This major change would require the availability of substantial numbers of internists or family practitioners at MTFs to perform comprehensive evaluations. It would also require better, more consistent explanations to MTF physicians about the purposes and procedures of the CCEP. It would require regional medical center physicians to provide adequate quality assurance of MTF work-ups and timely feedback to MTF providers.

On January 17, 1995, the DoD adopted these suggestions by setting goals that about 80% of patients would receive a definitive diagnosis at an MTF level. For some patients, this change has required specialty consultations at the MTF, as well as advice from an RMC physician. These changes necessitated an enhanced quality control role by the RMC physician and prompt, appropriate feedback to the MTF physician.

2.1.2.) Curtail diagnostic work-ups in patients not seriously disabled with minor complaints:

Initially, patients who do not accept their initial diagnosis could request a continued evaluation all the way through Phase II. The Committee recommends that diagnostic work-ups in patients not seriously disabled but with minor complaints should be curtailed. Alternatively, if a physician has made a definitive diagnosis and appropriate treatment has been given, the evaluation would be concluded.

On January 17, 1995, the DoD implemented the suggestions that referral to Phase II be made on the basis of the clinical judgment of the primary care physician, and patients were no longer permitted to self-refer to an RMC.

2.1.3.) Require additional efforts to provide more care at the primary care level:

The Committee encourages efforts to provide more care at the primary care level, because they will enhance the continuity of care and will foster the establishment of an ongoing therapeutic relationship.

2.1.4.) Continue referral of subgroups of patients whose illnesses are difficult to diagnose:

Patients whose illnesses are difficult to diagnose should continue to be referred to Phase II at an RMC. The decision to refer to Phase II should be based on the clinical judgment of the primary care physician, which, in turn, would be dependent on the clarity of the patient's diagnoses and the feasibility of the proposed treatment program at the MTF level. The DoD should continue its goal of enhanced accessibility of RMC physicians to allow regular consultations with MTF primary care physicians on patients with more complex diagnoses.

2.2.) Systematic Guidelines for Psychiatric Referrals and Adequacy of Psychiatric Resources:

2.2.1.) Develop explicit guidelines for the identification of Phase I patients who would benefit from a psychiatric evaluation:

CCEP physicians have noted the need for standardized guidelines for screening, assessing, evaluating, and treating patients. Such Phase I guidelines should be developed to help ensure adequate psychiatric resources for both the initial evaluation and long-term follow-up care.

2.2.2.) Alert primary care physicians about the high prevalence of psychiatric disorders:

Two methods that have been proposed by RMC physicians to expedite the scheduling of psychiatric evaluations would be (1) the more frequent use of civilian psychiatrists and (2) consideration of using Ph.D.-level psychologists, as well as psychiatrists, when necessary.

3.) SPECIFIC OBSERVATIONS OF AND RECOMMENDATIONS FOR THE IMPLEMENTATION OF THE CCEP:

3.1.) Analysis and Interpretation of the CCEP Results:

3.1.1.) Symptoms and diagnoses in the CCEP population:

3.1.1.1.) No evidence has been found that the DoD has been trying to avoid reaching a single unifying diagnosis:

The committee found no evidence that the DoD has been trying to avoid reaching a single "unifying" diagnosis when a plausible one was available. A "unifying" diagnosis is defined here as a single diagnosis that could explain most or all of a patient's symptoms.

3.1.1.2.) Signs and symptoms in many patients can be explained by well-recognized conditions:

One interpretation of the CCEP results is that the signs and symptoms in many patients can be explained by well-recognized conditions that are readily diagnosable and treatable. The committee concludes that this is a more likely interpretation than the interpretation that a high proportion of the CCEP patients are suffering from a unique, previously unknown "mystery disease."

3.1.1.3.) Provide more detailed information on specific diagnoses in future reports:

By providing more detailed information on specific diagnoses in its future reports, the DoD might help correct the impressions among the general public that exist about the high degree of prevalence of a "mystery disease" or a new, unique "Persian Gulf Syndrome."

3.1.1.4.) Investigate the diagnosis in patients with disability processing actions:

Disability processing actions in the Services' Physical Disability Processing Systems have been completed for 246 of the 10,020 CCEP patients. The DoD has not provided any data about their diagnoses or their reasons for medical separation from the military. The committee recommends that the DoD investigate the diagnoses in this group of patients in future reports, as well as whether or not the disorders could have been caused or exacerbated by service in the Persian Gulf.

3.1.1.5.) Don't view CCEP results as estimates of the prevalence of disability related to Persian Gulf service:

Many other individuals who served in the Persian Gulf have left active service and, hence, are not eligible for the DoD's CCEP. Some of these veterans may have disabilities related or unrelated to their service in the Persian Gulf, and those with disabilities might be more likely to have left active service. For these reasons, the CCEP results should not be viewed as estimates of the prevalence of disability related to Persian Gulf service.

3.1.2.) Evidence of a New, Unique Persian Gulf Syndrome:

3.1.2.1.) There is a lack of clinical evidence of a unique Persian Gulf Syndrome:

The committee agrees with DoD that there is currently no clinical evidence in the CCEP of a previously unknown, serious illness among Persian Gulf veterans. If there were a new or unique illness or syndrome among Persian Gulf veterans that could cause serious impairment in a high proportion of veterans at risk, it would probably be detectable in the population of 10,020 CCEP patients. On the other hand, if an unknown illness were mild or affected only a small proportion of veterans at risk, it might not be detectable in a case series, no matter how large.

3.1.2.2.) Share the entire CCEP data set with qualified researchers outside of the DoD:

The committee encourages the DoD's plan to share the entire CCEP data set with qualified researchers outside of the DoD who might be able to undertake the kind of research with the methodological sophistication that the identification of a new syndrome would require.

3.1.3.) Potential Relationship of Illnesses in CCEP Patients to Service in the Persian Gulf:

3.1.3.1.) Discuss the issue of causality explicitly and unambiguously in its future reports:

Physicians involved with the development and the administration of the CCEP have, in various public presentations, acknowledged that some CCEP patients have developed illnesses that are directly related to their service in the Persian Gulf. The recent DoD report on 10,020 CCEP participants, however, only touches on this issue indirectly. The committee encourages the DoD to discuss the issue of causality explicitly and unambiguously in its future reports. Such a discussion might help to alleviate the current climate of confusion and mistrust that exists among some Persian Gulf veterans and the general public.

3.1.3.2.) Determine the timing of the onset of disease:

The committee recommends that the DoD attempt to determine the timing of the onset of disease, especially for patients who have significant impairments. Review of military or civilian medical records that predate enrollment in the CCEP may provide contemporaneous documentation of the onset of symptoms in some patients, especially if the symptoms are serious. In addition, it is important to determine whether service in the Persian Gulf has contributed to the exacerbation of preexisting diseases in some CCEP patients.

3.1.4.) Comparison of the CCEP Population with Other Populations:

3.1.4.1.) Be cautious about comparison with other populations:

In its most recent report, the DoD compares the symptoms and diagnoses in the CCEP population with the symptoms and diagnoses in several community-based and clinically based populations. In the committee's view, interpretations based on comparisons with other populations should be made with great caution and only with the explicit recognition of the limitations of the CCEP as a self-selected case series. The CCEP was not designed to answer epidemiological questions, such as how the frequencies of certain diagnoses compare between the CCEP population and a control population. Instead, it was designed as a medical evaluation and treatment program. Indeed, the research aims of the CCEP do not appear to be stated explicitly, nor does there appear to be a concrete epidemiological study plan. Without research hypotheses, it is not possible to judge whether any particular comparison group is appropriate. Each individual population should be described to prevent confusion.

3.1.4.2.) It's difficult to establish causal relationships by relying on CCEP data alone:

It would be extremely difficult to establish causal relationships or to identify and characterize a new "Persian Gulf Syndrome" definitively by relying on data from the CCEP alone. The latitude permitted in the clinical examination program conflicts with the rigor necessary to answer an epidemiological question.

3.1.4.3.) Consider the CCEP data to have high clinical utility:

The CCEP data do have considerable clinical utility, and they could be used to address many important questions from a descriptive perspective. Many case series could be derived from these data. In addition, the results of the clinical exams could provide guidance in the selection of research questions and in the design of future epidemiological research. The CCEP findings could be used to generate epidemiological questions on other types of diseases that are much more frequent in the CCEP population, such as musculoskeletal diseases.

3.2.) Specific Medical Diagnosis:

3.2.1.) Psychiatric Conditions:

3.2.1.1.) Make patients aware of psychiatric conditions and their prevalence and morbidity:

Patients need to understand that psychiatric conditions and disorders are real diseases that cause real symptoms and that diagnoses are made with objective criteria and are not merely "labels" applied because physical abnormalities were not found. The CCEP patients, as well as their primary care physicians, also need to understand the prevalence of and the concomitant morbidity that result from psychiatric disorders in the general population (major depression, for example). Finally, the CCEP patients need to be aware that effective treatments that actually ameliorate symptoms exist for many of these disorders.

3.2.1.2.) Emphasize effects and diagnosis of psychosocial stressors:

In its future reports, the DoD is encouraged to emphasize that psychosocial stressors can produce physical and psychological effects that are as real and potentially devastating as physical, chemical, or biological stressors. The DoD should also emphasize that thorough efforts to diagnose psychiatric conditions in the CCEP population may lead to appropriate, successful treatments.

3.2.1.3.) Identify people with risk of developing depression or Post-Traumatic Stress Disorder (PTSD):

The committee is particularly concerned about the CCEP patients who have developed or who are at risk of developing major depression or PTSD. These people need to be identified and provided with some form of preventive intervention.

3.2.1.4.) Improve standardization of psychiatric evaluations:

The committee recommends that the DoD consider methods of improving the standardization of the psychiatric evaluations in the CCEP. The DoD should consider establishing detailed guidelines for the psychiatric evaluations and should attempt to obtain greater standardization of these evaluations among the various hospitals across the country. These guidelines could provide suggested procedures for the use of selected self-report instruments for the assessment of the most commonly diagnosed disorders, as well as procedures for more in-depth structured clinical interviews when indicated.

3.2.1.5.) Document and investigate the onset and course of symptoms and psychosocial stressors:

It would be especially important to document the onset and course of symptoms and to investigate their possible link with psychosocial stressors associated with mobilization and return home, as well as with service-related exposures in the Persian Gulf region. This assessment would require an additional set of questions to supplement the questionnaire currently used in Phase I of the CCEP. The thorough assessment of psychosocial stressors is essential information for treatment planning for patients with complex, chronic symptoms.

3.2.1.6.) Standardize neuropsychological evaluations:

Standardization of the neuropsychological evaluations is a related concern. The neuropsychological methods vary from pencil and paper testing at some sites to computer-administered testing at other sites. One method of achieving a better consensus is to convene a meeting attended by one psychiatrist and one neuropsychologist from each center to attempt to standardize their methods.

3.2.1.7.) Standardize classification and coding of diseases:

In addition to the standardization of psychiatric evaluations in the CCEP, the classification and coding of these diseases should also be standardized.

3.2.1.8.) Document headache categories differently:

The classification of different types of headaches into three separate categories may be consistent with ICD-9 coding rules, but the DoD should also report a special tabulation that combines all headaches into one group.

3.2.1.9.) Add explicit written instruction on medical record-keeping and coding:

More explicit written instructions could be added to the CCEP guidelines to help prevent the most frequent problems found in the medical record-keeping and coding. Committee comments about inconsistencies are mainly aimed at the quality control necessary for accurate reporting of summary data rather than at the quality of the medical care itself.

3.2.1.10.) Expand discussion of psychological stressors:

DoD should consider expanding discussion of the psychological stressors that were present during the Persian Gulf War.

3.2.1.11.) Utilize results of on-going studies to revise CCEP:

It is possible that the DoD will be able to use the results of on-going epidemiologic studies on psychiatric conditions to revise the CCEP, that is, to revise the standardized questionnaires or to add or delete targeted lab tests or specialty consultations. In addition, the CCEP clinicians may be able to utilize these results in the counseling and treatment of their patients. These results may also be useful for the DoD in its planning to minimize the effects of psychosocial stressors in future deployments through the use of preventive medicine interventions.

3.2.2.) Musculoskeletal Conditions:

3.2.2.1.) Provide more details of diagnostic categorization of musculoskeletal conditions:

The draft and final DoD reports on 10,020 CCEP patients do not provide adequate details for the IOM committee to make a thorough evaluation of the diagnostic categorization of musculoskeletal conditions. More explanation about the diagnostic aspects of these musculoskeletal conditions would be useful, for example, information on single-joint involvement versus multijoint conditions or articular versus non-articular conditions. In addition, details on disease severity and disease activity would be useful.

3.2.2.2.) Place more emphasis on musculoskeletal conditions:

The DoD and the DVA should consider placing more emphasis on research on musculoskeletal conditions, since these are the most prevalent disorders among the CCEP populations.

3.2.3.) Signs, Symptoms, and Ill-Defined Conditions:

3.2.3.1.) Clarify types of disorders included in the ICD-9 category:

The committee recommends that in future reports the DoD attempt to clarify the types of disorders that are included in the ICD-9 category of signs, symptoms, and ill-defined conditions (SSIDC). Individuals with these signs, symptoms, and ill-defined conditions should be evaluated in a rigorous manner, just as individuals with any other symptoms are evaluated.

3.2.4.) Infectious Diseases:

3.2.4.1.) Infectious disease is not a frequent cause of serious illness:

The IOM committee concludes that infectious diseases are not a frequent cause of serious illness in the CCEP population.

3.2.4.2.) Veterans are not likely afflicted with some previously unknown pathogen:

On the basis of the current evidence, it is unlikely that a significant proportion of Persian Gulf veterans are afflicted with some previously unknown pathogen that is evading the current diagnostic efforts.

3.2.5.) Chronic Fatigue Syndrome, Fibromyalgia, and Multiple Chemical Sensitivity:

3.2.5.1.) Estimating prevalence of chronic fatigue syndrome, fibromyalgia, and multiple chemical sensitivity is difficult:

The IOM committee's review of the CCEP protocol suggests that data on chronic fatigue syndrome (CFS), fibromyalgia (FM), and multiple chemical sensitivity (MCS) may have been collected by various diagnostic methods. For this reason, it is not possible to estimate the prevalence of these conditions from the CCEP data.

3.2.5.2.) Collect data using established diagnostic criteria for CFS and FM:

In the clinical evaluations, data should be collected by using established diagnostic criteria for CFS and FM.

3.2.5.3.) Established diagnostic criteria do not exist for MCS:

A widely accepted set of diagnostic criteria does not exist for MCS. Consequently, the medical evaluation in CCEP cannot be expected to diagnose the clinical syndrome of MCS.

3.2.5.4.) Include CFS, FM, and MCS in on-going and future epidemiological research studies:

If more is to be learned about the relationship between these disorders (CFS, FM, and MCS) and Persian Gulf service, they should be included among the epidemiological research studies that are ongoing or planned for the future.

3.2.5.5.) Continue thorough workup to diagnose sleep disturbances and fatigue:

Because of the thorough, systematic workup mandated in the CCEP, many disorders that could contribute to sleep disturbance and fatigue have been diagnosed. These diligent efforts to unmask occult medical problems that could substantially contribute to fatigue have been productive and should continue.

3.3.) Use of the CCEP Results for Education Improvements in the Medical Protocol and Outcome Evaluations:

3.3.1.) Use of the CCEP Results for Education:

3.3.1.1.) Continue public release of analysis results of the CCEP on an on-going, periodic basis:

The IOM committee encourages the DoD to continue to release its analysis of the results of the CCEP on an ongoing, periodic basis. Several audiences that would be interested in these results include active-duty members of the service, veterans, members of the U.S. Congress, the lay media, as well as military, DVA, and civilian medical and public health professionals. The CCEP medical findings would also be of interest to physicians in the DVA system and in the general community.

3.3.1.2.) Distribute CCEP findings to all primary care physicians at MTFs and RMCs:

The medical findings of the CCEP should be distributed promptly to all primary care physicians at the MTFs and RMCs. This would provide feedback on their diagnostic decision-making. Information on the frequencies of particular symptoms and their specific diagnoses made in the CCEP population could be useful, for instance, in developing a differential diagnosis for individual patients.

3.3.1.3.) Develop a more concise version of the DoD report for active-duty service personnel and veterans:

A more concise version of the DoD report on 10,020 patients, written in nontechnical language and with clearly stated conclusions, should be developed for a target audience of active-duty service personnel and veterans. If the DoD developed and distributed a fact sheet or newsletter aimed at Persian Gulf veterans, the information on the CCEP would be more accurate and more comprehensive than most reports in the general news media. This would also provide an additional opportunity to notify the readers about the availability of the medical exam in the CCEP, the hotline number, and the eligibility criteria.

3.3.1.4.) Develop a more comprehensive document describing potential exposures in more detail:

The DoD should also consider developing for clinical use in the CCEP a more comprehensive document that describes the many potential exposures in more detail. Any document that is prepared, however, must make clear what is known and what is unknown about the relationship between these stressors and the physical or psychological consequences.

3.3.2.) Use of the CCEP Results to Improve the Medical Protocol:

3.3.2.1.) Use CCEP examination results to improve standardization practices:

The DoD now has results on the examinations of more than 10,000 CCEP patients, which could be used to improve the standardized questionnaires, lab tests, and specialty consultations.

3.3.2.2.) Refine questions related to potential psychological stressors:

More refined questions related to potential psychological stressors could be added systematically to the Phase I medical history. The CCEP physicians might find this information useful in diagnosing and counseling their patients. In addition, it may be possible to identify patients who are at increased risk of psychological problems on the basis of their experiences in the war. Perhaps explicit questions on death exposure and other known risk factors could be added to the Phase I questionnaire.

3.3.2.3.) Determine if lab tests or specialty consultations should be added to Phase I:

The CCEP results should be analyzed to determine whether there are lab tests or specialty consultations that should be added systematically to Phase I to increase its diagnostic yield. Diseases that are diagnosed relatively frequently in Phase II may often be overlooked in Phase I. If such diseases could be identified, perhaps appropriate screening instruments could be added to Phase I.

3.3.2.4.) Compare and coordinate methods and clinical results of the CCEP and UCAP:

The DVA uses a protocol similar to that used in the CCEP called the Uniform Case Assessment Protocol (UCAP). The methods and clinical results of the CCEP and UCAP should be compared to coordinate and improve the two programs.

3.3.3.) Use of the CCEP Results for Patient Outcome:

3.3.3.1.) Perform targeted patient evaluations:

On the basis of more than 10,000 patient evaluations to date, RMC physicians could begin to perform a series of targeted patient evaluations. The most common diseases in the CCEP could be identified, and suggested approaches to patient treatment could be developed. Consensus guidelines for the treatment and counseling of CCEP patients who have the most common disorders could be useful for primary care physicians.

3.3.3.2.) Communicate successful treatment methods between RMCs:

If one RMC has had a lot of experience with a particular disease category and some measure of success in its treatment, the DoD could ensure that a description of their successful methods is communicated to the other MTFs and RMCs across the country.

3.3.3.3.) Review disorders among CCEP patients who have applied for disability payments or for medical discharge from the service:

The DoD could perform a review of the types and severities of the disorders among CCEP patients who have applied for disability payments or for medical discharge from the service. In addition, the final disposition of these cases could be evaluated, including the potential relationship between particular diseases and Persian Gulf service. The DoD could use the results of these disability determinations to predict which diseases are likely to be associated with the most impairment among CCEP patients in the future. The DoD could also use these results to develop rehabilitation and early intervention methods for impaired Persian Gulf veterans, such as the Specialized Care Centers (SCC). Another reason to analyze these disability claims would be to investigate possible preexisting risk factors for the development of the impairment. If such risk factors are identifiable, then targeted preventive medicine interventions could be planned for individuals participating in future overseas deployments.

3.3.4.) Specialized Care Center (SCC):

3.3.4.1.) The DoD has made serious efforts to develop an SCC program that has ambitious goals:

The IOM committee concludes that the DoD has made serious efforts to develop an SCC program with ambitious goals for a select group of seriously impaired military personnel. The committee's review should be considered preliminary, however, because it is based on one visit and it is still early in the development of the program.

3.3.4.2.) Provide multidisciplinary treatment modalities:

The SCC currently performs a thorough reevaluation of each patient's medical problems. SCC physicians should consider limiting the diagnostic role that they play to focusing on the incoming patients who have been very difficult to diagnose at the RMC level. Instead, the SCC should focus on providing multidisciplinary treatment modalities that are not readily available at the RMC level.

3.3.4.3.) Need for individualized follow-up and therapeutic regimens:

The need for individualized follow-up is crucial for the types of difficult patients who are likely to be treated at the SCC. Medical staff at the SCC will need to know whether a particular therapeutic plan is feasible at the patient's nearest MTF and whether long-term follow-up care can be performed. The primary care physician at the MTF needs to encourage continuous patient compliance with the carefully designed, individualized therapeutic regimens.

3.3.4.4.) Develop objective measure of functional status for follow-up evaluation:

The SCC physicians should develop a set of relatively objective measures of functional status for the follow-up evaluation. These could include (1) appropriate utilization of medical care, (2) appropriate use of medications or other methods to cope with symptoms, (3) general level of activities of daily living, (4) employment status, and (5) status of interpersonal relationships.

3.3.4.5.) Evaluate the SCC program itself:

The SCC program itself needs an evaluation component after several of its graduates have returned for their 6-month reevaluations. Several issues will need to be evaluated in light of the successes and barriers that the program has experienced, including eligibility criteria for patients; roles of the SCC in a diagnostic reevaluation of patients; successful continuity of care of patients, with shared responsibility by the SCC and MTFs; and the unique need for the SCC, beyond the usual standard of a tertiary care medical center.

3.3.4.6.) DoD has taken a serious approach to the treatment and rehabilitation of these patients in the SCC:

The committee believes that the DoD has taken a serious approach to the treatment and rehabilitation of these impaired patients who have treatable, chronic diseases.

3.3.4.7.) Investigate costs and benefits of the SCC program:

Because this program is very labor-intensive, it is probably very expensive on a per-patient basis. At the same time, the potential benefits for each patient could be high, if successful rehabilitation of serious, long-term impairment can be achieved. Subsequent evaluations of the SCC program should investigate its costs and benefits, if possible.

3.3.4.8.) Identify the most effective elements of the SCC program:

If the SCC program is successful in improving the health and functional status of its patients, perhaps the elements that are most effective in enabling the patients to cope with their symptoms could be identified. Perhaps some of these elements could be disseminated and integrated into existing MTF programs that are close to where CCEP patients live and work.

3.4.) Research Relevant to the CCEP:

3.4.1.) Epidemiological Research Relevant to the CCEP:

3.4.1.1.) Utilize on-going epidemiological studies for revising or improving the CCEP:

The results of on-going epidemiological studies may be useful for making revisions or improvements in the CCEP medical protocol itself, for example, to revise the standardized questionnaires or to add or delete targeted lab tests. The study results may also be useful in the counseling and treatment of CCEP patients.

3.4.1.2.) Acknowledge the serious limitations of the CCEP data for epidemiological purposes:

Data from individuals in the CCEP are also being used in some of these epidemiological studies. In these studies, the serious limitations of the CCEP data for epidemiological purposes that were previously identified must be kept in mind.

3.4.2.) Exposure Assessment Research Relevant to the CCEP:

3.4.2.1.) Investigate experiences of individuals in UICs with higher rates of CCEP participation:

The IOM committee encourages DoD to perform further investigations on the war and postwar experiences of individuals in the Unit Identification Codes (UICs) with higher rates of CCEP participation.

3.4.2.2.) Investigate exposures restricted to particular locations or special occupational groups:

The committee encourages the DoD to investigate exposures that were restricted to particular locations or special occupational groups, such as troops who had direct combat exposure. The types of symptoms and diseases in CCEP participants in these special groups and UICs could be analyzed and contrasted with the symptoms and diagnoses of CCEP participants in other units.

COMMITTEE ON THE DOD PERSIAN GULF SYNDROME COMPREHENSIVE CLINICAL EVALUATION PROGRAM

Gerard Burrow,* *Chair,* Dean, Yale University School of Medicine, New Haven, Connecticut

Dan Blazer,* Dean of Medical Education and Professor of Psychiatry, Duke University Medical Center, Durham, North Carolina

Margit Bleecker, Director, Center for Occupational and Environmental Neurology, Baltimore, Maryland

Ralph Horwitz, Chairman, Department of Internal Medicine, Yale University School of Medicine, New Haven, Connecticut

---

*Member, Institute of Medicine.

Howard Kipen, Associate Professor and Director, Occupational Health Division, Robert Wood Johnson Medical School, Piscataway, New Jersey
Adel Mahmoud,* Chairman, Department of Medicine, Case Western Reserve University and University Hospitals of Cleveland, Cleveland, Ohio
Michael Osterholm, State Epidemiologist, Minnesota Department of Health, Minneapolis, Minnesota
Robert Pynoos, Professor of Psychiatry, University of California at Los Angeles, Los Angeles, California
Anthony Scialli, Associate Professor, Department of Obstetrics and Gynecology, Georgetown University Medical Center, Washington, D.C.
Rosemary Sokas, Associate Professor of Medicine, Division of Occupational and Environmental Medicine, George Washington University School of Medicine, Washington, D.C.
Guthrie Turner, Chief Medical Consultant, Division of Disability Determination Services, State of Washington, Tummwater, Washington
Michael Weisman, Professor, Division of Rheumatology, University of California at San Diego Medical Center, San Diego, California

Staff
Michael A. Stoto, Director, Division of Health Promotion and Disease Prevention
Kelley A. Brix, Study Director
Deborah Katz, Research Assistant
Amy Noel O'Hara, Project Assistant
Donna D. Thompson, Division Assistant
Mona Brinegar, Financial Associate

Appendix E

Workshop on the Adequacy of the CCEP for Evaluating Individuals Potentially Exposed to Nerve Agents: Agenda and Speakers List

NATIONAL ACADEMY OF SCIENCES
INSTITUTE OF MEDICINE

December 3, 1996
Foundry Building FO-2004, Georgetown

AGENDA

10:00–10:15 Welcome/Purpose and Conduct of the Workshop
Dr. Dan Blazer, Chair, Committee on the Evaluation of the DoD Comprehensive Clinical Evaluation Program for Persian Gulf Veterans

10:15–12:00 Workshop Session I—Issues regarding the CCEP
Dr. Raymond Chung, *Origins/Background*
Dr. Charles Engel, *Mental Health*
Dr. Andrew Dutka, *Neurologic Conditions*
Dr. Timothy Cooper, *Pain*
Dr. Anthony Amato, *Neuromuscular Symptoms*
Dr. Kurt Kroenke, *Diagnostic Approach/ Generalized Symptoms*

12:00–1:00 Lunch in meeting room

1:00–2:45	Workshop Session II—Issues regarding organophosphates, anticholinesterases, and nerve agents Dr. Peter Spencer, *Neurotoxicology of organophosphates* Dr. Robert MacPhail, *Behavioral toxicology of organophosphates and pyridostigmine* Dr. Robert Gum, *Possible health effects in humans from low-level exposure to nerve agents* Dr. Bhupendra P. Doctor, *Endogenous detoxification of sarin*
2:45–3:00	Break
3:00–4:45	Workshop Session III—Issues regarding neurological testing protocols **Neurophysiological testing** Dr. Eva Feldman Dr. David Cornblath **Neurobehavioral and neurocognitive testing** Dr. Kent Anger Dr. Roberta White
4:45–5:00	Break
5:00–6:30	Workshop Session IV—Moderated Discussion Dr. Dan Blazer, *Moderator* Dr. Richard Johnson Dr. Arthur Asbury Dr. David Janowsky
6:30	Workshop adjourns

SPEAKERS

Anthony A. Amato, M.D.
University of Texas San Antonio
Department of Neurology and Medicine

W. Kent Anger, Ph.D.
Associate Director for Occupational Research and Health Promotion
Oregon Health Sciences University
Portland

Arthur Asbury, M.D.
Van Meter Professor of Neurology
Hospital of the University of Pennsylvania
Philadelphia

Col. Raymond Chung
Gulf War Health Center
Walter Reed Army Medical Center
Washington, DC

Lt. Col. Timothy W. Cooper, M.D.
Infectious Disease Service
74th Medical Group Hospital
Wright Patterson AFB, OH

David Cornblath, M.D.
Pathology Department
Johns Hopkins Hospital
Baltimore, MD

Bhupendra Doctor, M.D.
Director, Division of Biochemistry
Walter Reed Institute of Research
Washington, DC

Capt. Andrew J. Dutka, M.D.
Neurology Service
National Naval Medical Center
Bethesda, MD

Maj. Charles C. Engel, Jr., M.D.
Chief, Gulf War Health Center
Walter Reed Army Medical Center
Washington, DC

Eva Feldman, M.D., Ph.D.
Associate Professor
Department of Neurology
University of Michigan
Ann Arbor

Lt. Col. Robert Gum, M.D.
Chief, Chemical Casualty Care Office
U.S. Army Medical Research Institute of Chemical Defense
Aberdeen Proving Ground, MD

David Janowsky, M.D.
Department of Psychiatry
University of North Carolina Neurosciences Hospital
Chapel Hill

Richard Johnson, M.D.
Director, Department of Neurology
Johns Hopkins University School of Medicine
Baltimore, MD

Col. Kurt Kroenke, M.D.
General Internist
Uniformed Services University of Health Sciences
Bethesda, MD

Robert C. MacPhail, Ph.D.
Neurotoxicology Division
Environmental Protection Agency
Research Triangle Park, NC

Peter S. Spencer, Ph.D.
Director
Center for Research on Occupational and Environmental Toxicology
Oregon Health Sciences University
Portland

Roberta White, Ph.D.
Environmental Hazards Center
Department of Veterans Affairs Medical Center
Boston

Appendix F

Adequacy of the Comprehensive Clinical Evaluation Program: Nerve Agents*

RECOMMENDATIONS

The charge to the committee was to determine whether the Comprehensive Clinical Evaluation Program could adequately diagnose and treat possible health problems among service personnel who may have been exposed to low levels of nerve agents. The committee reviewed extensive clinical and research results regarding the effects of nerve agents. No evidence available to the committee conclusively indicated the existence of long-term health effects of low-level exposure to nerve agents. Because firm conclusions about these effects remain elusive, the committee reviewed information about the types of health effects that *might* exist as a result of exposure. Leading scientists presented information suggesting that the possible effects *might* include neurological problems such as peripheral sensory neuropathies and psychiatric problems such as alterations in mood, cognition, or behavior.

Recent reports suggesting a possible toxic synergistic effect following exposure to multiple agents known to influence cholinesterase activity will require extensive research to determine their significance (Haley and Kurt, 1997; Haley et al., 1997a,b; Lottie et al., 1993). The results of the research to date, however, did not appear to indicate any additional possible health effects should be considered by the committee other than those already identified.

---

*This appendix is excerpted from the Institute of Medicine report, *Adequacy of the Comprehensive Clinical Evaluation Program: Nerve Agents,* Washington, D.C.: National Academy Press, 1997.

The committee concluded that the CCEP continues to provide an appropriate screening approach to the diagnosis of disease. Most CCEP patients receive a diagnosis and 80% of participants receive more than one diagnosis. Although the types of primary diagnoses commonly seen in the CCEP involve a variety of conditions, 65% of all primary diagnoses fall into three diagnostic groups (1) psychological conditions; (2) musculoskeletal diseases; and (3) symptoms, signs, ill-defined conditions or a fourth group designated as "healthy." **However, in view of potential exposure to low levels of nerve agents, certain refinements in the CCEP would increase its value.** These refinements are viewed as part of a natural evolution and improvement process and, therefore, need not be applied retrospectively. The committee does encourage rapid implementation in order to provide the benefits of an improved system to new enrollees.

The committee recommends improved documentation of the screening used during Phase I for patients with psychological conditions such as depression and posttraumatic stress disorder (PTSD). The DoD (DoD, 1996) reported that depression and PTSD account for a substantial percentage of those receiving a diagnosis of a psychological condition. In addition, if there are long-term health effects of nerve agent exposure, it is possible that these effects could be manifested as changes in mood or behavior. The committee will be conducting an in-depth examination of the adequacy of the CCEP as it relates to stress and psychiatric disorders at a later time; however, because of the increased importance of ensuring that all possibilities are thoroughly checked, better documentation in this area is encouraged. Primary physicians could use any of a number of self-report screening scales, but consistent use of the same scale across facilities would ensure consistent results.

The committee recommends improved documentation of neurological screening done during both Phase I and Phase II of the CCEP. Concern about nerve agent exposure as well as the number of nonspecific, undiagnosed illnesses among CCEP patients makes documentation of neurological screening extremely important. CCEP patients are referred to neuromuscular specialists if they have complaints of severe muscle weakness, fatigue, or myalgias lasting for at least 6 months that significantly interfere with activities of daily living. These patients are evaluated by board-certified neurologists who have subspecialty training in neuromuscular disease. Based on the description of the tests administered and examinations conducted, the committee finds that the CCEP is sufficient to ensure that no chronic, well-established neurological problem is being overlooked. The documentation of the use of these tests and procedures, however, could and should be improved. Such improvements would engender confidence that neurological examinations and treatments across facilities are comparable.

Given the importance of thorough neurological and psychiatric screening, **the committee recommends that Phase I primary physicians have ready access to a referral neurologist and a referral psychiatrist.** As mentioned earlier, patients are referred to neuromuscular specialists if they have complaints of severe muscle weakness, fatigue, or myalgias lasting for at least 6 months that significantly interfere with activities of daily living. Appropriate psychiatric referrals could include those with chronic depression that is treatment-resistant, an unexplained, persistent complaint of memory problems, or significant impairment secondary to behavioral difficulties, such as not being able to maintain productive work due to behavioral abnormalities. While patients referred for Phase II consultations with a neurologist or psychiatrist are cared for adequately, it is sometimes difficult for the primary physician to determine whether or not a referral is appropriate. In such instances, the physician tends to refer more frequently than not. It may be that, if the primary care physician had neurological and psychiatric consultations readily available, referral decisions could be made more easily and appropriately.

The committee recommends that physicians take more complete patient histories, particularly regarding personal and family histories, the onset of health problems, and occupational and environmental exposures. While there currently is grave concern about exposure to nerve agents during deployment in the Persian Gulf, other factors have an affect on psychological and neurological disorders. Patients can perform below expectations on neuropsychological tests for a number of reasons. In clinical assessments, therefore, it is important to rule out alternative causes of impairment. In addition, current and past exposures to occupational and environmental toxicants are important. Detailed histories are a valuable tool in identifying the etiology of a patient's problems.

The committee recommends that, to the extent possible, predeployment physical examinations given to members of the armed forces should be standardized among the services. The lack of uniform baseline information about service members makes diagnosis and treatment of postdeployment problems more difficult. To the extent that adequate baseline information is unavailable, physicians must rely on self-reporting. Adequate predeployment physical examinations, standardized across services, could prove an important tool for both clinical assessment and structured research.

The committee recommends that DoD increase the uniformity of CCEP forms and reporting procedures across sites. The CCEP system would benefit from increased consistency and the knowledge that each service is collecting and using the same information. Currently, each branch of service and each facility use different forms to complete examinations, tests, and referrals. Increasing the consistency of such forms and procedures would provide a more reliable picture of the care given to patients in the CCEP. As was stated in the

1996 report on the Health Consequences of Service During the Persian Gulf War, it is extremely important to create a uniform, continuous, and retrievable medical record. In addition, the 1996 report stated that the information should be collected according to standardized procedures and maintained in a computer-accessible format (IOM, 1996b). The committee concurs with those findings.

For each patient, the physician should provide written evidence that all organ systems were evaluated. The CCEP primary care physicians examine patients, and, if there are problems requiring additional expertise, the patients are referred to specialists. This is standard medical practice used across the United States. It would be appropriate, however, for the CCEP primary care physicians to document that their evaluations covered all organ systems. The committee is not recommending the use of new or sophisticated testing mechanisms. It is reinforcing the importance of the components of the basic medical examination. This increased documentation could be completed by noting the organ systems evaluated and whether each was normal or abnormal. For those listed as abnormal, additional information could be provided.

The committee strongly urges the DoD to offer group education and counseling to soldiers and their families concerned about exposure to toxic agents. Following the revelation by the DoD of possible exposure to nerve agents due to the destruction of the munitions dump at Khamisiyah, approximately 20,000 service personnel received a letter from the DoD stating that their units were in the vicinity during the demolition. Each recipient was encouraged to contact an 800 number if he or she was experiencing health problems believed to be a result of service in the Persian Gulf. Given this revelation, there may be a heightened sense of insecurity and concern among Persian Gulf veterans and their families about possible exposure to nerve agents. Risk communication is an important clinical activity. Family and group counseling can address heightened concerns about exposure as well as other issues. Such an approach provides an appropriate public health mechanism for imparting information and addressing concerns and should be made available to all Persian Gulf veterans.

Although it is beyond the scope of the charge to this committee to determine whether low-level exposure to nerve agents causes long-term health effects, the committee believes strongly that this is an important research area that ought to be pursued. Most of the literature regarding health effects of exposure to nerve agents (i.e., sarin and cyclosarin) addresses exposures high enough to cause clinically observable effects. These clinical effects are well documented and include miosis, blurred vision, nausea, vomiting, muscular twitching, weakness, convulsions, and death. Little known research has been conducted regarding the long-term health effects of low levels of exposure to these nerve agents. The application of findings from research on organophosphate pesticide exposure to the area of nerve agent exposure has limitations. However, even in such pesticide studies, long-term health effects have been documented only for acutely poisoned individuals—that is, persons with immediate clinical symptoms.

The committee emphasizes that the CCEP is *not* an appropriate vehicle for scientifically assessing questions about long-term health effects of low levels of exposure to nerve agents. *The CCEP is a clinical treatment program, not a research protocol.* It is important, therefore, not to attempt to use the findings of the CCEP to answer research questions. Those questions must be addressed through rigorous scientific research.

The committee notes that the CCEP could be useful in identifying promising directions for separate research studies. Examinations of the health effects—if any—of various wartime exposures have been hampered by poor information about the level of exposure and an inability to identify the individuals who may have been exposed. It is often difficult to retrospectively estimate exposure levels. However, information about where individuals were and when they were there could be combined with data regarding the presence of an exposure to develop surrogate measures. These surrogate measures could then be linked to health information and used to examine potential associations between exposures and health effects.

Although data from the CCEP cannot be used to *test* for associations, it can be combined with other information to help identify areas for future research. For example, the DoD identified approximately 20,000 service people belonging to units that were within a 50-kilometer radius of Khamisiyah at the time of the munitions demolition. Examining the health records of these people may yield insights into whether those who participated in the CCEP (or a similar program administered by the VA) have different illnesses or patterns of illnesses than do CCEP participants outside the 50-kilometer radius. More detailed discrimination of proximity to Khamisiyah (e.g., within 20 kilometers or within the units directly responsible for the munitions destruction) may provide additional information.

It is important, however, to understand the limitations of such comparisons. The results cannot be taken as research findings and generalized to the entire population of those deployed to the Persian Gulf. Active-duty military personnel participating in the DoD health registry may be either more or less healthy than other nonparticipants on active duty. CCEP comparisons on this self-selected group of patients should not be used to draw conclusions about the entire population of Persian Gulf veterans.

More broadly, the committee notes that information that helps to identify where individuals were in the Persian Gulf and when they were there will also facilitate research into potential service-related health problems. This information is currently needed to address the question of who might have been exposed to nerve agents and who could be part of the (unexposed) comparison groups necessary for epidemiological studies. Such information could also be used to more quickly and easily identify the exposed and unexposed groups that would be required to assess any future concerns regarding this or other exposures.

Generating geographical and temporal information for all 700,000 people who served in the Persian Gulf would be an immense endeavor. It would not be prudent to undertake such a task without first thoroughly understanding the effort required to complete it. It would, however, be appropriate to take steps now to identify and preserve records that could assist in the generation of such a database in the future. Records-based information is intrinsically superior to personal recollections, especially several years after the fact.

COMMITTEE ON THE EVALUATION OF THE DoD COMPREHENSIVE CLINICAL EVALUATION PROGRAM

Dan G. Blazer,* *Chair,* Dean of Medical Education and Professor of Psychiatry, Duke University Medical Center, Durham, North Carolina

Margit L. Bleecker, Director of the Center for Occupational and Environmental Neurology, Baltimore, Maryland

Evelyn J. Bromet, Professor, Department of Psychiatry, State University of New York at Stony Brook, Stony Brook, New York

Gerard Burrow,* Dean, Yale University School of Medicine, New Haven, Connecticut

Howard Kipen, Associate Professor and Director, Occupational Health Division, Robert Wood Johnson Medical School, Piscataway, New Jersey

Adel A. Mahmoud,* Chairman, Department of Medicine, Case Western Reserve University and University Hospitals of Cleveland, Cleveland, Ohio

Robert S. Pynoos, Associate Professor of Psychiatry and Dean of the Trauma Psychiatry Service, University of California at Los Angeles, Los Angeles, California

Guthrie L. Turner, Chief Medical Consultant, Office of Disability Determination Services, State of Washington, Tummwater, Washington

Michael Weisman, Professor, Division of Rheumatology, University of California at San Diego Medical Center, San Diego, California

Staff

Lyla M. Hernandez, Study Director

Sanjay S. Baliga, Research Associate

---

*Member, Institute of Medicine.

David A. Butler, Senior Program Officer
Donna M. Livingston, Project Assistant
James A. Bowers, Project Assistant
Kathleen R. Stratton, Director, Division of Health Promotion and Disease Prevention
Constance M. Pechura, Director, Division of Neuroscience and Behavioral Health

Appendix G

Workshop Agendas and Speakers Lists

WORKSHOP ON DIFFICULT-TO-DIAGNOSE AND ILL-DEFINED CONDITIONS

Green Building, Washington, D.C.
March 3, 1997

AGENDA

8:30–8:45	**Welcome and Introduction** Dan G. Blazer, M.D., Chair, Committee on the Assessment of the DoD Comprehensive Clinical Evaluation Program
8:45–10:00	**Chronic Fatigue Syndrome** *Description/ Diagnosis and Treatment Description/Diagnosis* Dedra S. Buchwald, M.D. *Treatment* Nelson Gantz, M.D. *Q & A*
10:00–10:15	**BREAK**

10:15–11:30	**Fibromyalgia** *Definition/Diagnosis* Frederick Wolfe, M.D. *Treatment* Robert Simms, M.D. *Q & A*
11:30–12:30	**Multiple Chemical Sensitivity** *Description, Diagnosis, and Treatment* Howard Kipen, M.D., M.P.H. *Q & A*
12:30–1:30	**Lunch in Meeting Room**
1:30–2:00	**Difficult to Diagnose and Ill-Defined Conditions—A Discussion of the Issues** Daniel J. Clauw, M.D.
2:00–2:30	**What are the Criteria for a Good Screening Instrument** Penelope M. Keyl, Ph.D.
2:30–3:30	**Department of Defense Presentation** *Signs, symptoms, and ill-defined conditions* Maj Charles Magruder *Fibromyalgia and Chronic Fatigue Syndrome in the CCEP* Lt Col Tim Cooper *Interpretation of CCEP Data: Diagnostic and Treatment Approaches to Date* COL Kurt Kroenke
3:30	**ADJOURN WORKSHOP**

SPEAKERS

Dedra Stefanie Buchwald, M.D.
University of Washington
Seattle, WA

Daniel J. Clauw, M.D.
Georgetown University
Washington, DC

Lt Col Tim Cooper
74th Medical Group Hospital
Wright-Patterson AFB, OH

Nelson M. Gantz, M.D., F.A.A.C.P.
Polyclinic Hospital
Harrisburg, PA

Penelope M. Keyl, Ph.D.
Johns Hopkins University
Baltimore, MD

Howard Kipen, M.D., M.P.H.
Environmental and Occupational Health Sciences Institute
Piscataway, NJ

COL Kurt Kroenke
Uniformed Services University of Health Sciences
Bethesda, MD

MAJ Charlie Magruder
Deployment Surveillance Team
Falls Church, VA

Maj Edwin C. Matthews
59th Medical Wing Hospital
Lackland AFB, TX

Robert Simms, M.D.
Boston University School of Medicine
Boston, MA

Frederick Wolfe, M.D.
The Arthritis Center
Wichita, KS

WORKSHOP ON STRESS AND PSYCHIATRIC DISORDERS

Arnold and Mabel Beckman Center
Irvine, CA
May 22, 1997

AGENDA

8:00 **Welcome and Introduction**
Dan G. Blazer, M.D., Chair
Committee on the Evaluation of the CCEP

8:15–10:15 **Stressors**
General Stressors
Carol Aneshensel, Ph.D.
Military Stress(including combat and Gulf War specific)
Charles Engel, M.D.
Stress and its Effects on the Endocrine and the Immune Systems
Firdaus Dhabhar, Ph.D.
Discussion

10:15–10:30	**BREAK**
10:30–11:00	*Substance Abuse* Walter Ling, M.D.
11:00–12:00	Department of Defense *Description of Diagnostic Process/Protocol Data Presentation* Michael Roy, M.D.
12:00–1:00	**LUNCH**
1:00–1:30	Department of Defense *Specialized Care Center* Charles Engel, M.D.
1:30–3:30	*Posttraumatic Stress Disorder (PTSD)* David Foy, Ph.D. *Diagnosing Depression in a Primary Care Setting* John D. Wynn, M.D. *Subthreshold Depressions: Clinical, Familial, and Sleep EEG Validation* Hagop Akiskal, M.D. *Discussion*
3:30	**WORKSHOP ENDS**

SPEAKERS

Hagop Akiskal, M.D.
University of California
San Diego, CA

Carol Aneshensel, Ph.D.
University of California
Los Angeles, CA

Firdaus Dhabhar, Ph.D.
The Rockefeller University
New York, NY

MAJ Charles Engel, M.D., MC
Walter Reed Army Medical Center
Washington, DC

David Foy, Ph.D.
Pepperdine University
Malibu, CA

Walter Ling, M.D.
University of California
Los Angeles, CA

MAJ Michael Roy, M.D., MC
Walter Reed Army Medical Center
Washington, DC

John D. Wynn, M.D.
University of Washington
Seattle, WA

Appendix H

Outline of the CCEP Medical Protocol

FORM REQUIREMENTS

At the MTF level, the CCEP record should include all CCEP forms and relevant medical data to the program.

Blank forms included with this guide supersede previous editions of these forms and are intended to be used with the new CCEP.

All individual forms will be complete and legible.

Forms forwarded to NMIMC and maintained in the participant record shall be in the following order:

Phase I completed:

MTF Phase I Diagnosis Form
Patient Questionnaire
Provider-Administered Symptom Questionnaire
Information Release Form
Declination/Completion Form

Phase II completed:

RMC Phase II Diagnosis Form
Declination/Completion Form

MEDICAL PROTOCOLS

The CCEP is based upon a thorough clinical evaluation which emphasizes comprehensive and continuous primary care. The local MTF primary care provider maintains responsibility for patient evaluation and care throughout the CCEP process.

Medical Treatment Facility (Phase I)

Phase I will consist of a comprehensive history and medical evaluation with completion of Phase I questionnaires and related forms. The examination, both in content and quality, should parallel an inpatient admission work-up. The Phase I examination will include a complete medical history including: family, occupation, social (including tobacco, alcohol, and drug use), exposure to possible toxic agents, psychosocial condition and review of symptoms. The provider will specifically inquire about the symptoms listed on the CCEP Provider-Administered Patient Questionnaire. A comprehensive medical evaluation, with focused attention to the patients' symptoms and health concerns, should be conducted.

Individuals who, after completing MTF Phase I evaluations, do not have a clearly defined diagnosis which explains their symptoms should be reviewed by the CCEP-designated physician for further evaluation and consultations needed and/or for referral to the RMC.

Phase II level evaluations are performed only after complete clinically indicated evaluations (including appropriate specialty consultations) are conducted at the MTF and the RMC.

Phase I Laboratory Tests
CBC
U/A
SMA-12

Regional Medical Center (Phase II)

Phase II evaluations consist of the following laboratory tests, consultations, and as necessary, symptom-specific examinations. Elements of the Phase II evaluation may be accomplished by the local MTF as needed in the comprehensive evaluation of the Phase I patient in order to obtain a definitive diagnosis.

Phase II Laboratory Tests

CBC
Sedimentation rate (ESR)
C-Reactive protein
Rheumatoid factor
ANA
Liver function
CPK
Urinalysis
TB skin test (PPD) with controls
Chest X-ray
Hepatitis serology
HIV testing
VDRL
B12 and folate
Thyroid function tests

Phase II Consults

(if not accomplished at MTF level)
Dental: Dental only if participant's annual screening not done
Infectious disease
Psychiatry: With physician-administered instruments:
Structured Clinical Interview for DSMIII-R
(SCID) (delete modules for mania and psychosis)
Clinician-Administered PTSD Scale (CAPS)

Neuropsychological Testing: Only as indicated by psychiatry consult

SYMPTOM-SPECIFIC EXAMINATIONS

The RMC CCEP physician ensures that Phase II patients with the following undiagnosed symptoms receive the tests and consultations listed below.

Diarrhea
GI consult
Stool for O and P
Stool leukocytes
Stool culture
Stool culture
Stool volume
Colonscopy with biopsies
EGD with biopsies and aspiration

Muscle Aches/ Numbness
EMG/NCV

Chronic Fatigue
Polysomnography and MSLT

Chronic Cough/SOB
Pulmonary consult
Pulmonary function
Tests with exercise and ABG
Methacholine challenge
If PFTs are normal, consider bronchoscopy with biopsy/ lavage

Abdominal
GI consult
EGD with biopsy/ aspiration
Colonscopy with biopsy
Abdominal ultrasound
UGI series with small bowel FT
Abdominal CT scan

Memory Loss
(Only if verified by psych evaluation)
MRI—head
Lumbar puncture
Neuro consult
Neuro psych testing

Chest Pain/ Palpitations
ECG
Exercise stress test
Holter monitor

Headache
MRI—head
LP (glucose protein, cell count, VDRL, oligoclonal myelin, basic protein, pressure)
Neuro consult

Vertigo/Tinnitus
Audiogram
ENG
BAER

Skin Rash
Dermatology consult
Consider biopsy

Reproductive Concerns
Urology consult
GYN consult

Appendix I

Screening Instruments for Substance Abuse

CAGE

1. Have you tried to *cut down* on your drinking or use?
2. Do you get *annoyed* by others' comments about your drinking or use?
3. Do you ever feel guilty about your drinking or use?
4. Do you ever take an eye opener in the morning to get going?

Brief *MAST*

1. Do you feel you are a normal drinker?
2. Do friends or relatives think you are a normal drinker?
3. Have you ever attended a meeting of Alcoholics Anonymous (AA)?
4. Have you ever lost friends or girlfriends/boyfriends because of drinking?
5. Have you ever neglected your obligations, your family, or work for 2 or more days in a row because you were drinking?
6. Have you ever had delirium tremens (DTs), severe shaking, or seen things that weren't there after heavy drinking?
7. Have you ever gone to anyone for help about your drinking?
8. Have you ever been in a hospital because of drinking?
9. Have you ever been arrested for drunk driving or driving after drinking?
   (Pokotny et al., 1972)

T-ACE

T TOLERANCE: How many drinks does it take to make you feel high?

A Have people ANNOYED you by criticizing your drinking?

C Have you ever felt you ought to CUT down on your drinking?

E EYE OPENER: Have you ever had a drink first thing in the morning?

Two or more positive responses indicate that the woman is likely to have an alcohol problem (Sokol et al., 1989).

TWEAK

T TOLERANCE: How many drinks can you hold?

W Have close friends or relatives WORRIED or complained about your drinking in the past year?

E EYE OPENER: Do you sometimes take a drink in the morning when you first get up?

A AMNESIA: Has a friend or family member ever told you about things you said or did while you were drinking that you could not remember?

K(C) Do you sometimes feel the need to CUT down on yourdrinking?

A 7-point scale is used to score the test. The tolerance question scores 2 points if the woman reports she can hold more than five drinks without falling asleep or passing out. A positive response to the WORRIED question scores 2 points, and a positive response to the last three questions scores 1 point each. A total score of 2 or more points indicates that the woman is likely to have an alcohol problem (Russel et al., 1993).

AUDIT

1. How often do you have a drink containing alcohol?
2. How many drinks containing alcohol do you have on a typical day when you are drinking?

4. How often during the last year have you found that you were unable to stop drinking once you started?
5. How often during the last year have you failed to do what was normally expected from you because of drinking?
6. How often during the last year have you needed a first drink in the morning to get yourself going after a heavy drinking session?
7. How often during the last year have you had a feeling of guilt or remorse after drinking?
8. How often during the last year have you been unable to remember what happened the night before because you had been drinking?
9. Have you or someone else been injured as the result of your drinking?
10. Has a relative, friend, doctor, or other health worker been concerned about your drinking or suggested you cut down?